RAND NATIONAL DEFENSE RESEARCH INSTITUTE

Pre-Deployment Stress, Mental Health, and Help-Seeking Behaviors Among Marines

Carrie M. Farmer, Christine Anne Vaughan, Jeffrey Garnett,
Robin M. Weinick

Prepared for the Office of the Secretary of Defense and the Defense Centers of Excellence for Psychological Health and Traumatic Brain Injury

For more information on this publication, visit www.rand.org/t/rr218

Library of Congress Cataloging-in-Publication Data is available for this publication.

ISBN: 978-0-8330-8382-1

Published by the RAND Corporation, Santa Monica, Calif.

Preface

The Marine Corps Operational Stress Control and Readiness (OSCAR) program is designed to embed mental health personnel within deploying Marine Corps units and enable marines in officer and senior noncommissioned officer (NCO) roles to extend the reach of these mental health personnel by providing early recognition and intervention for marines exhibiting signs of stress. Toward this goal, select officers and senior NCOs attend a training course that provides instruction on OSCAR principles, as well as the appropriate recognition, intervention, and referral of marines with potential mental health problems. The Defense Centers of Excellence for Psychological Health and Traumatic Brain Injury (DCoE) has asked RAND to evaluate the OSCAR program.

Our evaluation of the OSCAR program has four main components: (1) longitudinal pre- and post-deployment surveys of marines from OSCAR-trained and non–OSCAR-trained battalions, (2) longitudinal pre- and post-deployment surveys of OSCAR team members, (3) semistructured interviews with commanding officers of battalions that received OSCAR training, and (4) focus groups with battalion leaders, health care providers, and chaplains who received OSCAR training prior to deployment. This report describes our findings from the pre-deployment, or baseline, survey of marines from OSCAR-trained and non–OSCAR-trained battalions. The results in this report are among the first to shed light on the pre-deployment mental health status of marines, as well as the social resources they draw on in coping with stress and their attitudes about seeking help for stress-related problems.

The results of this report will be of particular interest to national policymakers within the Department of Defense (DoD) working to maintain the mental health of service members and should also be useful for health policy officials within the U.S. Department of Veterans Affairs (VA). Researchers working to understand the relationship between pre-deployment characteristics of service members and post-deployment mental health problems will also be interested in these findings.

This research was sponsored by DCoE and conducted within the Forces and Resources Policy Center of the RAND National Defense Research Institute, a federally funded research and development center sponsored by the Office of the Secretary of Defense, the Joint Staff, the Unified Combatant Commands, the Navy, the Marine

Corps, the defense agencies, and the defense Intelligence Community under Contract W74V8H-06-C-0002. For more information on the RAND Forces and Resources Policy Center, see http://www.rand.org/nsrd/ndri/centers/frp.html or contact the director (contact information is provided on the web page).

Contents

Figures

Tables

Summary

Background

U.S. military forces have been engaged in extended conflicts in Iraq and Afghanistan since 2001. During that time, service members have faced extended deployments and exposure to combat or other stressful situations. While most military personnel cope well with these stressors, many experience difficulties handling stress at some point, and some experience mental health problems as a consequence. The prevalence of posttraumatic stress disorder (PTSD) among returning U.S. service members is estimated at 5–20 percent, with variations in this estimate due to differences in how the population is defined and which measures are used (Ramchand et al., 2011). The literature suggests that certain populations of service members may be at higher risk for deployment-related mental health problems, including those with greater combat exposure (Seal et al., 2009; Hoge, Auchterlonie, and Milliken, 2006). Numerous programs have been developed to assist service members with deployment-related stress and mental health problems; a recent RAND report estimated that the U.S. Department of Defense (DoD) alone funds over 200 such programs.

One such program, the Marine Corps Operational Stress Control and Readiness (OSCAR) program, is intended to provide mental health support to marines by (1) embedding mental health personnel within Marine Corps units and (2) increasing the capability of officers and senior NCOs to improve the early recognition and intervention of marines exhibiting signs of stress. To this end, select officers and senior NCOs at the battalion and company levels attend a one-day training course that delivers instruction on OSCAR principles, as well as the recognition, intervention, and referral of marines with potential stress injuries. Our research team is evaluating the impact of the OSCAR program. This report presents the results of the first phase of our evaluation study.

Purpose of This Report

This report presents findings from a pre-deployment survey of 2,620 marines scheduled for deployment to Afghanistan or Iraq. We developed the survey primarily as a means of gathering baseline information to support our evaluation of the OSCAR program. However, it also provides unique information about marines' mental health prior to deployment, as well as their attitudes toward stress and seeking help for mental health issues. Though a great deal of research has examined mental health and stress-related concerns among military service members following deployment, this report contributes to the nascent literature on the mental health status of service members prior to deployment. This report also contributes to an understanding of the magnitude of mental health problems and associated vulnerabilities that are present prior to service members' first deployment, as roughly half of the marines in this study had never deployed as of the time of the survey.

Specifically, the pre-deployment survey asked questions about four main topics:

- mental health burden (i.e., mental health status and high-risk drinking behavior)
- prior exposure to traumatic events
- resources for coping with stress
- attitudes toward coping with stress and seeking help.

Methods

The survey was administered as part of a study designed to determine whether marines in battalions that received OSCAR training fared better in terms of stress and mental health–related outcomes from pre- to post-deployment relative to marines in battalions that did not receive OSCAR training. The study was quasi-experimental, in that the two survey groups were not created by random assignment but by comparing two naturally occurring groups that were similar at baseline. The study included a survey both before and after deployment; this report describes the findings from the pre-deployment survey.

The pre-deployment survey was conducted in person with marines from seven battalions (three service support battalions and four infantry battalions) preparing for a combat deployment to Afghanistan. The survey was fielded in group settings to 2,975 marines on base between March 2010 and December 2011. A total of 2,620 marines completed the survey, representing a cooperation rate of 88.1 percent.

The survey included questions about sociodemographic and service history characteristics, any lifetime history of traumatic events, current stress, mental health status, high-risk drinking, the use of social resources to cope with stress and potential mental health problems, and attitudes toward stress response and recovery. When available, well-validated measures of these constructs were used. When well-validated measures did not exist, we borrowed relevant questions from other surveys or created original questions to assess the construct.

Since our survey sample was not a random sample, the survey data were weighted to match the sociodemographic and service history characteristics of the larger population of marines who deployed to Iraq or Afghanistan in 2010 or 2011. This study design affords stronger inferences regarding the mental health status and high-risk drinking behavior within this population in advance of deployment.

Key Findings

Mental Health Burden

The 2,620 marines in the survey sample had high rates of positive screens for current major depressive disorder (MDD) (12.5%) and high-risk drinking (25.7%). Rates of these problems were three to four times higher among enlisted marines than officers based on the officers surveyed. Rates of high-risk drinking were particularly high among junior enlisted marines (rank E1–E3), with roughly a third (33.1%) reporting high-risk alcohol use. Rates of these problems did not vary significantly by type of battalion or deployment history.

To place these findings in context, we compared them to estimates of the prevalence of these problems from nationally representative datasets, which found that the rate of current depression among adult males in the U.S. general population was 6.4 percent. Data from a nationally representative survey, the National Epidemiological Survey on Alcohol and Related Conditions (NESARC), indicate that, adjusting for the age distribution of our sample of marines, 16.1 percent of adult males in the U.S. population engage in high-risk drinking behavior, as measured by the cutoff applied in our study. Of particular interest, even those marines in our sample who had never deployed had higher rates of positive screens for current major depressive disorder (12.4%; 95% confidence interval [CI] [10.4%, 14.4%]) and high-risk drinking behavior (25.2%; 95% CI [21.8%, 28.7%]) relative to adult males in the U.S. general population.

Previous Exposure to Traumatic Events

The survey asked marines about exposure to potentially traumatic events during their lifetime. On average, marines in the sample reported that they had experienced 3.9 (95% CI [3.6, 4.1]) types of potentially traumatic events over their lifetime (out of a possible 17 types of events). The types of events most frequently reported were motor vehicle accidents (66.4%); the sudden, unexpected death of a loved one (45.4%); and physical assault (38.0%). Just over one-quarter (28.2%) of marines reported having experienced a natural disaster, 4.7 percent of marines reported having experienced a sexual assault, and 19.2 percent of marines reported having experienced combat.

The total number of potentially traumatic events experienced varied significantly by rank, battalion type, and deployment history. A significantly higher number of events was reported by marines of rank E4–E9 (mean [M] = 4.30, 95% CI [3.82, 4.77]) relative to marines of rank E1–E3 (M = 3.55, 95% CI [3.36, 3.74]) and officers (M = 2.89, 95% CI [2.28, 3.49]); by marines in infantry battalions (M = 4.18, 95% CI [3.89, 4.48]) relative to marines in service support battalions (M = 3.55, 95% CI [3.35, 3.75]); and by marines who had previously deployed to Iraq or Afghanistan (M = 5.21, 95% CI [4.31, 6.11]) relative to marines who had not previously deployed (M = 3.39, 95% CI [3.24, 3.54]).

To put these findings in context, we compared them to findings from the National Comorbidity Survey (NCS), a nationally representative survey in which respondents were asked to indicate which of several types of potentially traumatic events they had directly experienced during their lifetime (Kessler et al., 1995). In comparison to adult males in the general population, a higher proportion of marines in our study reported having experienced different types of potentially traumatic events. This finding might be expected given that roughly half of the marines in our study had previously deployed to Iraq or Afghanistan and would likely have had exposure to several types of potentially traumatic events during their deployment. However, even among the subset of marines in our study who had never deployed, the rates of having experienced potentially traumatic events were higher than those of adult males in the U.S. general population: Only (11.1%) of the NCS general male population (compared with 37.4 percent of the sample of marines who had never deployed) had directly experienced a physical assault; 18.9 percent of the general male population had experienced a natural disaster (compared with 26.8 percent of marines who had never deployed); and 0.7 percent of the general male population had experienced a sexual assault (compared with 5.0 percent of marines who had never deployed).

The Use of Resources for Coping with Stress

The survey also asked respondents about what kinds of social or other resources they turn to for help in coping with stress. Marines were asked whether they had ever talked with, or recommended that a buddy talk with, a number of types of individuals that could be used as resources for dealing with stress.

Most marines reported having used (79.3%) or recommended (88.7%) one or more of the following resources for dealing with stress: a buddy, leader, chaplain, corpsman, or unit medical officer. The most common type of resource cited by respondents when dealing with their own stress was a buddy (71.9%). Similarly, the majority of marines reported recommending a buddy as a resource to others in need of help with stress (84.0%). After buddies, leaders were the next most popular resource for helping oneself (49.7%) and for recommending to a buddy (67.7%).

We found significant differences between marines who had previously deployed to Iraq or Afghanistan at least once and marines who had never deployed in the types of resources recommended to a buddy for help with stress. Marines who had previously deployed were significantly more likely than those who had never deployed to report having recommended any type of resource for help (ever-deployed: 91.0%; never-deployed: 88.0%), as well as every specific type of resource aside from a buddy: leaders (ever-deployed: 71.9%; never-deployed: 66.4%), corpsmen (ever-deployed: 44.5%; never-deployed: 34.6%), chaplains (ever-deployed: 70.9%; never-deployed: 57.1%), and unit medical officers (ever-deployed: 35.9%; never-deployed: 25.8%). In notable contrast, there were no differences between those who had previously deployed and those who had never deployed in the use of resources for help with one's own stress.

Attitudes Toward Coping with Stress and Perceived Levels of Support

Marines were asked about their attitudes toward stress-related issues, as well as their perceptions of available support. Our research team created original items to measure respondents' attitudes about several issues related to stress and how to cope with it. These included: their self-perceived readiness; the ability to handle their own stress and help a peer handle his or her stress; the perceived efficacy of their peers and leaders in resolving their own stress problems and helping the respondent to resolve his or her stress problems; the extent to which they believe the responsibility to handle stress problems is shared by all marines; and the perceived stigmatization of or support for seeking help for stress problems at the level of the respondent's peers, leaders, unit, and the Marine Corps overall.

Overall, marines reported positive attitudes toward their own and others' abilities to cope with stress. On a five-point scale, with "1" representing the least positive attitude, "3" being neutral, and "5" representing the most positive attitude, respondents registered a mean score of 4.01 (95% CI [3.97, 4.05]).

We found significant differences in attitudes toward stress response and recovery by rank. Junior enlisted marines (E1–E3) reported the least positive attitudes toward stress response and recovery (M = 3.92, 95% CI [3.86, 3.97]) compared to E4–E9 marines (M = 4.06, 95% CI [4.00, 4.13]) and officers (M = 4.12, 95% CI [4.02, 4.22]).

We also found a significant differences by deployment history. Marines who had never deployed endorsed significantly less-positive attitudes toward stress response and recovery (M = 3.98, 95% CI [3.94, 4.03]) compared to marines who had deployed once or more (M = 4.10, 95% CI [4.04, 4.16]). There were no differences by battalion type.

Respondents also reported on a five-point scale that they perceived moderate levels of support for help-seeking (M = 3.12, 95% CI [3.06, 3.18]). We did not find significant differences in the perceived support for help-seeking by rank, battalion type, or deployment history.

Conclusions and Recommendations

Pre-Deployment Mental Health Burden

The results suggest that, even prior to deployment, marines face a substantial mental health burden. They are also more likely than their counterparts in the general population to have been exposed to traumatic events. Potential mental health problems may be even greater among junior enlisted marines. Therefore, marines would benefit from a greater emphasis on pre-deployment screening and assessment to facilitate problem resolution prior to deployment.

Recommendation 1: Consider implementing programs to identify and address mental health and alcohol use problems prior to deployment.

Recommendation 2: Investigate the relationship between the pre-deployment mental health burden, experiences while in theater, and the likelihood of developing longer-term mental health problems.

Recommendation 3: Target prevention and treatment efforts toward junior enlisted marines.

Recommendation 4: Consider additional training in combat and operational stress for junior enlisted marines.

Attitudes Toward Coping with Stress and Seeking Help and the Use of Help-Seeking Resources

The marines in our sample generally expressed positive attitudes toward stress response and recovery, and they perceived moderate levels of support for seeking help related to mental health problems. However, some stigma around mental health problems was apparent.

Recommendation 5: Provide training in stress recognition and response to all marines.

Recommendation 6: Continue to make multiple resources for help available to accommodate varied preferences.

Concluding Observation

Even prior to a deployment, marines face a mental health burden higher than that of the general U.S. population and also report higher levels of exposure to trauma. These results suggest that pre-deployment mental health deserves greater attention, from both DoD program planners and researchers seeking to understand service members' mental health and well-being across the deployment cycle.

Acknowledgments

We gratefully acknowledge the support of our current and previous project monitors, Mr. Yoni Tyberg, CAPT Anthony Arita, CAPT John Golden, and Col Christopher Robinson, and staff at DCoE, particularly Dayami Liebenguth. We also acknowledge the support of our points of contact in the Marine Corps Combat and Operational Stress Control office, Ms. Patricia Powell and MSgt Michael O'Brien. We appreciate the comments provided by our reviewers, Dr. Matthew Chinman and Dr. William Nash. Their constructive critiques were addressed, as part of RAND's rigorous quality assurance process, to improve the quality of this report. We acknowledge the support and assistance of David Adamson, Joshua Breslau, Craig Martin, Claude Setodji, Reema Singh, Anna Smith, and Phoenix Voorhies in the preparation of this report. We are also grateful to the marines who participated in our survey for their time and to our points of contact at each base for their time and support.

Abbreviations

AUDIT-C	Alcohol Use Disorders Identification Test-Consumption
BRFSS	Behavioral Risk Factor Surveillance Survey
CI	confidence interval
COSC	Combat and Operational Stress Continuum
DCoE	Defense Centers of Excellence for Psychological Health and Traumatic Brain Injury
DMDC	Defense Manpower Data Center
DoD	Department of Defense
DSM-IV	Diagnostic and Statistical Manual of Mental Disorders, 4th Edition
HSPC	Human Subjects Protection Committee
J-MHAT 7 OEF	Joint Mental Health Advisory Team 7 to Operation Enduring Freedom
LEC	Life Events Checklist
LL	lower limit
M	mean
MDD	major depressive disorder
MOS	military occupational specialty
NCO	noncommissioned officer
NCS	National Comorbidity Survey
NESARC	National Epidemiological Survey on Alcohol and Related Conditions

OEF	Operation Enduring Freedom
OIF	Operation Iraqi Freedom
OSCAR	Operational Stress Control and Readiness
PCL	PTSD Checklist
PCL-C	PCL-Civilian Version
PDHA	Post Deployment Health Assessment
PHQ-2	Patient Health Questionnaire-2
POC	point of contact
PTSD	posttraumatic stress disorder
UL	upper limit
VA	U.S. Department of Veterans Affairs

CHAPTER ONE

Introduction

Despite the drawdown of troops in Afghanistan and the end of the war in Iraq in 2011, U.S. military forces have been engaged in extended conflicts over the past decade, causing service members and their families to face extended deployments and exposure to combat or other stressful situations. While most military personnel and their families cope well with these stressors, many experience difficulties handling stress at some point. Over the past several years, the Department of Defense (DoD) has implemented numerous programs that address these issues by building resilience, preventing stress-related problems, and identifying and treating such problems. To understand the impact these programs have on service members and their families, the RAND Corporation has been engaged in an effort to catalog (Weinick et al., 2011) and evaluate DoD-sponsored programs addressing psychological health.

One such program, the Marine Corps Operational Stress Control and Readiness (OSCAR) program (1) embeds mental health personnel within Marine Corps units and (2) increases the capacity of officers and senior noncommissioned officers (NCOs) to improve the early recognition of and intervention for marines exhibiting signs of stress. Toward this goal, select officers and senior NCOs attend a one-day training course that delivers instruction in OSCAR principles, as well as the recognition, intervention, and referral of marines with potential mental health problems.[1] RAND is conducting an evaluation of the OSCAR program that includes four components: (1) longitudinal pre- and post-deployment surveys of marines from OSCAR-trained and non–OSCAR-trained battalions; (2) longitudinal pre- and post-deployment surveys of OSCAR team members; (3) semistructured interviews with commanding officers of battalions that received OSCAR training; and (4) focus groups with battalion leaders, health care providers, and chaplains who had received OSCAR training prior to deployment. A report on the overall findings from this evaluation, along with conclusions and recommendations for the OSCAR program, will be forthcoming.

This report presents findings from one component of our evaluation: a predeployment survey of marines. Using this survey, we collected information about the

---

[1] Additional information about the OSCAR program is available in Appendix A.

mental health status of marines, how marines cope with stress-related concerns, and their attitudes about seeking help. While the mental health of service members returning from combat deployment has been widely studied, the mental health burden and help-seeking behaviors and attitudes of service members *prior* to a combat deployment are not well understood. Therefore, the findings we report here will be useful to policymakers interested in the psychological health of military service members and are a valuable contribution to the nascent literature on the pre-deployment stress, mental health, and help-seeking behaviors and attitudes of active-duty marines.

Purpose and Organization of This Report

This report presents findings from the pre-deployment survey of marines. While we developed this survey to examine the effect of the OSCAR program on various outcomes for marines, it also provides unique information about marines' attitudes toward combat and operational stress, the burden of stress and mental health problems, and help-seeking behaviors. Though there have been studies elsewhere reporting on some of these issues among service members, this survey is the first to describe mental health status and help-seeking behaviors among marines.

In Chapter Two of this report, we present background information on previous efforts to assess the prevalence of mental health problems among service members, population characteristics that may be associated with these problems, and gaps in the scientific literature regarding the mental health of marines. Chapter Three details the methods we used to conduct the pre-deployment survey and analyze the survey data. Chapter Four presents our findings. Chapter Five presents conclusions and recommendations based on those findings.

This report also includes three appendices. Appendix A contains information about the OSCAR program and RAND's evaluation of the program. Appendix B contains additional technical detail about our methods. Results from the pre-deployment survey that were not of sufficient substantive importance to warrant inclusion in the main body of the report can be found in Appendix C.

CHAPTER TWO

Background

This report provides information about the mental health of a large group of marines prior to deployment, as well as risk factors that may be associated with potential mental health problems. Despite the large number of studies about the mental health of service members in the post-deployment period, the contribution of pre-deployment characteristics to mental health problems that occur during and after a deployment remains poorly understood. In this chapter, we review what is known about stress and mental health problems among service members, highlight gaps in existing knowledge, and discuss how our analysis is intended to help fill those gaps.

The Prevalence of Mental Health Problems and Alcohol Misuse in Military Populations

There is a large and growing literature on the mental health of service members and how it is affected by deployment and combat experiences. While the prevalence of mental health problems varies across studies, partially due to variations in research methods, there is a strong consensus that mental health problems, in particular posttraumatic stress disorder (PTSD), depression, and alcohol misuse, impose a large burden on the military population.

Posttraumatic Stress Disorder

PTSD, a disorder that develops in response to a traumatic event, is perhaps the primary mental health concern for service members who have served in Iraq and Afghanistan. According to the *Diagnostic and Statistical Manual of Mental Disorders* (DSM-IV), diagnostic criteria for PTSD include 17 symptoms organized into the following three clusters: the re-experiencing of the event (e.g., repeated, disturbing memories of the event), the avoidance of reminders of the event and numbing (e.g., efforts to avoid reminders of the trauma, diminution of interest or involvement in activities that were of interest prior to the trauma), and hyperarousal (e.g., hypervigilance) (American Psychiatric Association, 1994). PTSD is associated with significant functional impairment, and some with the disorder develop chronic mental health disabilities (Kessler, 2000).

A recent review by the Institute of Medicine concluded that the current prevalence of PTSD among service members who had deployed in support of Operation Iraqi Freedom (OIF) or Operation Enduring Freedom (OEF) falls somewhere between 13 percent and 20 percent (Institute of Medicine, 2012). In the few studies that have examined PTSD specifically within OEF/OIF marines, prevalence estimates have spanned a wider range. One study found that 10.8 percent of marines who had deployed to Iraq or Afghanistan screened positive for post-deployment PTSD (Phillips et al., 2010). Another study of infantry marines who had deployed to Iraq found that the prevalence of probable PTSD ranged from 12.2 percent to 19.9 percent, depending on the criteria employed to define probable PTSD (Hoge et al., 2004). Yet another study reported that 25 percent of previously deployed OEF/OIF marines screened positive for PTSD, although this estimate was based on a very small sample size (Eisen et al., 2012).

In short, myriad studies of the prevalence of PTSD among OEF/OIF service members have been conducted, and they report a wide range of prevalence estimates (Ramchand et al., 2010; Sundin et al., 2010). This variation is primarily due to differences in how the population was sampled and how prevalence was measured (e.g., whether the data were collected anonymously or as part of an "on-the-record" screening, whether the data corresponded to a symptom checklist or formal diagnosis, when the assessment was conducted).

Most studies of the mental health of previously deployed OEF/OIF service members have been conducted on convenience samples that are not representative of the population of previously deployed OEF/OIF service members (Ramchand et al., 2008). As combat exposure is an important predictor of PTSD, the extent to which the sampled population's exposure to combat varies will have a strong effect in the observed prevalence estimates. For example, studies of infantry marines (such as Hoge et al., 2004) are likely to find higher rates of PTSD than those of service support marines, who often have less direct combat experience.

Studies of random samples of service members that adjust for these differences are likely to produce more-robust prevalence estimates. One study that was conducted on a random sample of the population of previously deployed OEF/OIF service members and adjusted for differences between the sample and the population in several sociodemographic and service history characteristics found that 13.8 percent of respondents met the criteria for a probable diagnosis of PTSD (Schell and Marshall, 2008). A similarly designed study whose sample closely resembled the population of previously deployed OEF/OIF service members in a wide array of sociodemographic and service history characteristics yielded a comparable prevalence estimate, with 15.8 percent of the sample screening positive for probable PTSD (Vaughan et al., 2011).

Because all U.S. service members are asked to complete a Post Deployment Health Assessment (PDHA), studies that utilize data from this assessment may contain the most representative sample of the previously deployed OEF/OIF force (Hoge, Auchterlonie, and Milliken, 2006; Milliken, Auchterlonie, and Hoge, 2007). However, because of the potential for service members to experience negative consequences if they screen positive for mental health problems upon their return from deployment, such as a delay in their reunion with family members or adverse effects on their military career, service members may underreport mental health symptoms in "on-the-record" screenings such as the PDHA (Sundin et al., 2010). Comparing the rates of PTSD obtained through anonymous versus "on-the-record" screenings shows roughly twice the proportion of respondents screened positive for PTSD when the assessment was conducted anonymously (McLay et al., 2008; Warner et al., 2011a).

Variations in the instruments and cut-off scores used to identify PTSD lead to different prevalence estimates. Studies that impose stricter criteria for defining cases of PTSD (e.g., defining PTSD caseness as having both a PTSD Checklist [PCL] score > 50 and meeting DSM-IV criteria) report a lower prevalence (Ramchand et al., 2010; Thomas et al., 2010). In one study that systematically varied the strictness of the criteria for determining probable PTSD in a sample of active-component soldiers who had returned from deployment to Iraq or Afghanistan three months prior to the assessment, estimates of the prevalence of probable PTSD ranged from 6.3 percent to 20.7 percent, corresponding to the most- and least-strict criteria, respectively (Thomas et al., 2010).

Finally, the timing at which mental health assessments are conducted with respect to the service member's return from deployment may also account for some of the variability in prevalence estimates of PTSD across studies. While only a few studies have evaluated changes in the prevalence estimates of mental health problems as a function of time since return from deployment, these have found that the prevalence of PTSD increases during the months following return from deployment (Bliese et al., 2007; Milliken, Auchterlonie, and Hoge, 2007; Thomas et al., 2010).

Depression

Depression, one of the most disabling psychiatric disorders, has also been identified as a major concern among veterans of the wars in Iraq and Afghanistan (Tanielian and Jaycox, 2008; Institute of Medicine, 2010). Symptoms of depression include depressed mood, loss of interest or pleasure, changes in weight or appetite, insomnia or hypersomnia, psychomotor agitation or retardation, fatigue or loss of energy, feelings of worthlessness or guilt, impaired concentration, and recurrent thoughts of death or suicidal ideation (American Psychiatric Association, 1994). To meet the diagnostic criteria for depression, an individual must have at least five of these symptoms nearly every day during the same two-week period, and one of the symptoms must be depressed mood or loss of interest or pleasure.

Monitoring the prevalence of depression is one of the goals of the Joint Mental Health Advisory Team 7 to OEF (J-MHAT 7 OEF). The J-MHAT report is distinctive because it provides estimates of the prevalence of mental health problems in theater as opposed to after return from deployment. A recent study by J-MHAT found that about 5.3 percent of soldiers and 3.3 percent of marines (each from a sample that included ranks E1–E4, NCOs, and officers) scored above the threshold for clinically significant depression on a self-report screening test (J-MHAT 7 OEF, 2011).

A review of studies that examined rates of depression among the OEF/OIF force found that estimates ranged from two to ten percent (Ramchand et al., 2008). The sources of variability in the prevalence estimates of PTSD described above likely also account for variability in the prevalence estimates of depression. Two studies with samples that were broadly representative of the previously deployed OEF/OIF force produced estimates of probable major depressive disorder (MDD) of 13.7 percent (Schell and Marshall, 2008) and 15.7 percent (Vaughan et al., 2011). In one study of active-component soldiers who had returned from Iraq or Afghanistan three months prior to the assessment, the stringency of criteria employed to determine probable major depressive disorder was varied to elucidate the impact of definitional differences on prevalence estimates. Estimates of the prevalence of probable major depressive disorder ranged from 8.3 percent to 16.0 percent, corresponding to the most- and the least-strict criteria, respectively (Thomas et al., 2010).

Alcohol Use

Similar to studies of the prevalence of PTSD and depression among previously deployed OEF/OIF service members, studies of the rates of alcohol misuse yield widely varying estimates. In light of the known adverse implications of a positive screen for alcohol misuse on service members' military careers (e.g., disciplinary action and possible separation), collecting data on alcohol misuse anonymously is essential to obtaining accurate estimates of its prevalence in active-duty military populations. When interpreting findings from the existing literature on alcohol use among service members, it is important to note that this literature uses a variety of definitions and metrics of alcohol misuse. Among soldiers who deployed to Iraq, anonymous assessments of alcohol misuse using a two-item screening question[1] conducted approximately three months after returning from deployment yielded rates of alcohol misuse of 25 percent (Wilk et al., 2010) and 12.4 percent (Thomas et al., 2010). One study that anonymously assessed the alcohol use of OEF/OIF service members within one year of their return from deployment identified 39 percent of the sample as meeting criteria for probable alcohol abuse, defined as a score of five or greater on the Alcohol Use Disorders Identification Test–Consumption (AUDIT-C) (Eisen et al., 2012). Another study that assessed alcohol use anonymously using a two-item screening question one year after return from

[1] The screening questions were: "In the past 4 weeks, have you used alcohol more than you meant to?" and "In the past 4 weeks, have you felt you wanted or needed to cut down on your drinking?"

deployment to Iraq found that 9.9 percent of soldiers in the active component screened positive for alcohol misuse (Thomas et al., 2010). Among male OEF/OIF veterans seen in the Veterans Administration health care system, the rate of alcohol misuse (AUDIT-C score ≥ 5) was 21.8 percent, roughly twice the rate of alcohol misuse among male veterans who did not deploy in support of OEF/OIF (10.5%) (Hawkins et al., 2010).

Some of the studies cited above indicate high rates of alcohol misuse among previously deployed OEF/OIF service members (e.g., more than one in five service members). However, it is important to note that one of the only studies to compare alcohol use and binge drinking across previously deployed OEF/OIF male veterans and their civilian male counterparts in the U.S. general population, with adjustment for age and race/ethnicity, found only one difference in their drinking behaviors: civilians consumed a higher average quantity of alcohol on the days that they drank relative to their peers who had previously deployed for OEF/OIF (Ramchand et al., 2011). Thus, although the rate of alcohol misuse among males who had previously deployed for OEF/OIF suggests the need for policies and interventions to address alcohol use problems in this population, the magnitude of these problems does not appear to be any greater in this population than among civilian peers of the same gender, age, and race/ethnicity.

Very few studies have examined the prevalence of alcohol misuse specifically among marines. In one study that reported rates of alcohol misuse within one year of redeployment from Iraq or Afghanistan by branch of service (Eisen et al., 2012), 45 percent of marines screened positive for alcohol misuse, which was similar to the rate of alcohol misuse (based on AUDIT-C score ≥ 5) observed among soldiers (47%) but nearly twice as high as the rates of alcohol misuse found among airmen (26%) and sailors (26%). However, there were only 25 marines in this study, thereby calling into question the stability of this estimate. Another study in which infantry marines were anonymously surveyed about potential alcohol misuse after returning from deployment to Iraq found that 35.4 percent reported having used alcohol more than they had intended and 29.4 percent reported having wanted or needed to cut down on drinking (Hoge et al., 2004). By contrast, the same questions about alcohol misuse were endorsed by 24.2 percent and 20.6 percent, respectively, of infantry soldiers who had deployed to Iraq during the same time frame (Hoge et al., 2004). More studies are needed to shed light on the prevalence of alcohol misuse among marines.

Deployment-Related Factors That May Affect Mental Health

To ensure that efforts to prevent and treat mental health problems and alcohol misuse reach the most vulnerable individuals, it is important to identify the service-related characteristics and experiences of service members that confer increased risk of mental health and alcohol use problems. Several service-related characteristics and experiences have been studied, including rank and deployment-related experiences (e.g., combat trauma exposure).

Rank

Little research has examined mental health differences associated with differences in rank. Rank has a large impact on several aspects of deployment experience, including required roles, duties, and combat conditions. Rank may also be a proxy for educational attainment, with officers having higher educational attainment than enlisted service members, and lower-ranking members of the military are likely to be younger than higher-ranking members.

In general, studies have documented a higher risk of PTSD among previously deployed OEF/OIF service members of enlisted rank relative to officers, even after adjusting for multiple potentially confounding sociodemographic and service history characteristics (Lapierre, Schwegler, and LaBauve, 2007; Maguen et al., 2010; Schell and Marshall, 2008; Smith et al., 2008). Of particular interest, one study that examined the adjusted odds of developing new-onset PTSD from pre- to post-deployment within each branch of service found that, although lower rank conferred increased vulnerability to new-onset PTSD among soldiers, sailors, and airmen, it did not significantly increase the risk of new-onset PTSD among marines (Smith et al., 2008). In contrast, another study that evaluated the contribution of rank to post-deployment PTSD among enlisted marines who had deployed in support of OEF/OIF found that junior enlisted marines (E1–E3) had significantly higher adjusted odds of screening positive for post-deployment PTSD than did NCOs of ranks E4 and E5 (Phillips et al., 2010; Smith et al., 2008). More research is needed to further elucidate the association between rank and PTSD in marines.

A similar pattern of results has been found regarding depression: Enlisted service members have been identified as having a greater risk of depression than officers (Lapierre, Schwegler, and LaBauve, 2007; Maguen et al., 2010; Schell and Marshall, 2008). Very little research has examined the relationship between rank and alcohol misuse; one study failed to find a significant association between these variables (Ramchand et al., 2011).

Deployment-Related Experiences

Many studies have assessed the impact of characteristics of the deployment experience on mental health problems, including deployment duration, the number of previous deployments, and exposure to combat-related trauma (e.g., witnessing death, maimed service members or civilians, prisoners of war, etc.) during deployment. Studies tend to converge on the conclusion that the most important aspect of deployment with respect to mental health outcomes is exposure to combat trauma (Ramchand et al., 2010; Schell and Marshall, 2008; Smith et al., 2008). Service members in combat units who deployed in support of OEF/OIF report frequent exposure to combat-related traumatic events, particularly those deployed to Iraq. For instance, a study of members of Army and Marine Corps combat infantry units surveyed after returning from deployment found that the prevalence of being attacked or ambushed was 58 percent among soldiers deployed to Afghanistan, 89 percent among soldiers deployed to Iraq, and 95 percent among marines deployed to Iraq (Hoge et al., 2004). While traumatic events experienced during combat have been shown to confer increased risk of PTSD in OEF/OIF veterans (Hourani, Yuan, and Bray, 2003; Phillips et al., 2010; Ramchand et al., 2010; Schell and Marshall, 2008; Seal et al., 2009; Smith et al., 2008; Vaughan et al., 2011), there is also evidence that exposure to combat-related trauma elevates the risk for depression (Schell and Marshall, 2008) and alcohol use problems (Ramchand et al., 2011; Wilk et al., 2010).

Gaps in Existing Knowledge

The literature to date highlights the role of combat-related trauma in post-deployment mental health problems. However, this focus on combat-related traumatic exposure has inadvertently obscured the potential influence of pre-deployment traumatic events and mental health problems on post-deployment mental health problems. While little is known about service members' pre-deployment trauma history and mental health burden, two studies found that violence exposure prior to combat is a statistically significant predictor of post-deployment PTSD even after adjusting for combat experiences (Phillips et al., 2010; Clancy et al., 2006). Another study demonstrated stronger adverse effects of combat trauma exposure on post-deployment PTSD among service members who reported higher levels of functional impairment prior to deployment (Wright et al., 2011). Similarly, the Millennium Cohort Study, which was designed to prospectively evaluate the long-term health of service members, found that pre-deployment mental health problems were associated with higher rates of post-deployment PTSD (Sandweiss et al., 2011). Collectively, these findings underscore the need to consider pre-deployment vulnerabilities, such as lifetime trauma history and associated mental health problems, in understanding of the range of influences on post-deployment mental health problems.

Based on our review of this literature, we identified several gaps and designed a secondary analysis of our pre-deployment survey data from the OSCAR program evaluation to help fill these gaps. Specifically, we took advantage of our large sample of marines preparing to deploy to Iraq or Afghanistan in 2010 or 2011 (N = 2,620), roughly half of whom had never previously deployed to Iraq or Afghanistan, to accomplish the following goals:

- Describe the prevalence of mental health and alcohol use problems among marines preparing to deploy to Iraq or Afghanistan.

- Assess pre-deployment factors that might influence service members' response to deployment stress, such as prior mental health problems, lifetime history of traumatic events, rank, and history of deployment.
- Document the social resources marines use to cope with the stresses of deployment, as well as their attitudes toward coping with stress.

Our analysis is intended to address gaps in the literature by

- providing data on a large, representative sample of marines: *Most available research on mental health problems among marines who have deployed to Iraq or Afghanistan is based on small or unrepresentative samples.* Little research has been well suited to examining the prevalence of mental health problems specifically among marines who have deployed to Iraq or Afghanistan. Much of the extant data on marines have been based on small or unrepresentative samples (Eisen et al., 2012; Phillips et al., 2010), which limits confidence in population-level inferences drawn regarding the magnitude of mental health problems among marines who have deployed to Iraq or Afghanistan. Our sizable sample of marines preparing to deploy (N = 2,620) was weighted to match the sociodemographic and service history characteristics of the larger population of marines who deployed to Iraq or Afghanistan in 2010 or 2011. This study design affords stronger inferences regarding the rates of probable PTSD and MDD, as well as high-risk drinking, within this population in advance of deployment.
- identifying more reliable prevalence estimates of mental health and alcohol misuse problems among marines: *On-the-record assessments of mental health problems in military populations have been shown to underestimate the magnitude of mental health problems.* Our data may be especially advantageous for elucidating the true extent of mental health problems in this population, as they were collected exclusively for research purposes by a nonmilitary entity rather than through mental health assessments conducted by the military and included in the service member's military record (i.e., "on-the-record" screenings). Assessments of mental health symptoms conducted "off-the-record," under the promise of confidentiality, such as the findings reported here, should yield prevalence estimates of mental health and alcohol misuse problems that more closely correspond to the true prevalence of these problems in the population.
- focusing on the mental health status of marines before a deployment and identifying potential pre-deployment risk factors: *The majority of studies on military service members' mental health have focused on the contribution of combat trauma exposure to post-deployment mental health.* There is a gap in the literature with regard to the magnitude of mental health problems and associated vulnerabilities that are present prior to service members' first deployment and combat exposure. The focus on the influence of exposure to combat trauma on post-deployment

mental health implies that some proportion of service members enter the military in good psychological health and leave it "broken" by the combat they experience during deployment. This study is well positioned to test this assumption, which has rarely been examined, because roughly half of our survey sample had never previously deployed as of the time our data were collected. Our overall study is designed to capitalize on this opportunity to quantify and compare pre- and post-deployment mental health problems, and this report specifically assesses the frequency of potentially traumatic events experienced in marines' entire lifetimes, even before deployment. In addition to examining how mental health problems vary by deployment history, we examined differences in mental health problems by rank and type of battalion (infantry versus service support).

- describing marines' attitudes toward stress and help-seeking behaviors: *Little is known about service members' attitudes toward and behaviors used to cope with stress.* One of the main goals of the OSCAR program is to increase the likelihood that a marine who experiences significant mental health problems during or after deployment will receive appropriate mental health treatment. Understanding marines' attitudes toward seeking help for stress and mental health problems prior to implementation of the OSCAR program provides a necessary baseline for making this assessment. We therefore sought to increase our understanding of these attitudes and the social resources used to cope with the stresses of deployment. Numerous studies have assessed service members' mental health problems, but much less is known about the approaches they take to address mental health and stress problems. This report describes a snapshot of the coping behaviors and attitudes in place prior to OSCAR training by assessing several types of behaviors that marines have taken in response to stress and their attitudes toward dealing with stress.

CHAPTER THREE

Methods

The pre-deployment survey of marines that is the focus of this report was part of a quasi-experimental study designed to determine whether marines in OSCAR-trained battalions fare better in terms of stress and health-related outcomes from pre- to post-deployment relative to marines from non–OSCAR-trained battalions. The overall evaluation was longitudinal and included a post-deployment survey to assess the effects of the OSCAR program. Results of the complete longitudinal evaluation will be presented in a subsequent report.

Sampling

We followed a two-stage sampling procedure. First, we sampled seven Marine Corps battalions, including three service support battalions and four infantry battalions. Our contacts in the Combat and Operational Stress Continuum (COSC) office identified eligible battalions, which included active-duty or reserve units that were preparing for a combat deployment to Iraq or Afghanistan in 2010 or 2011.

Second, we sampled companies from within the battalions. We sampled between three and five companies from each of the four infantry battalions. For the first two infantry battalions, companies were randomly sampled within the battalion. Because random sampling proved very logistically challenging to implement, we sampled all available companies from the two remaining infantry battalions.

For two of the composite service support battalions, we also attempted to recruit all available companies in the battalion. From the third composite service support battalion, we sampled only two companies (one from the main battalion, one from another battalion that was augmenting the main battalion) because this recruitment fully met our target sample size.

Participation in the survey was further restricted to marines of rank O6 (Colonel) or lower. Additional information about the sampling strategy is available in Appendix B.

All marines of rank O6 (Colonel) or lower within each company were sampled for survey participation, and the cooperation rate was 88.1 percent.[1] The final sample size was 2,620 marines.

Procedures

Pencil-and-paper surveys were administered in person in a group setting on base prior to deployment. Respondents were informed that participation was voluntary and written informed consent was obtained. Additional information about the procedures is available in Appendix B.

Measures

The pre-deployment survey was designed to provide baseline assessments of short- and longer-term outcomes that OSCAR was expected to affect and the sociodemographic and service history characteristics that we planned to include in adjusted analyses of OSCAR's effect on the targeted outcomes post-deployment. The short-term outcomes were those that OSCAR would be expected to affect within a few months (e.g., attitudes toward stress response and recovery and help-seeking behavior). The longer-term outcomes were those that OSCAR would be expected to affect within six to 12 months, such as symptoms of PTSD and MDD.

When available, well-validated measures of the outcomes of interest, described below, were included in the pre-deployment survey. For several outcomes, however, measures used in previous studies had not been extensively validated or did not exist. In these instances, we borrowed relevant items from surveys and, when this was not possible, we developed new survey items to capture the construct of interest. Below we describe the measures included on the survey.

[1] 2,975 marines had the opportunity to participate in the survey, with 2,620 marines completing the survey and 355 marines declining to participate. The denominator for a true response rate calculation is unknown, as there may have been other marines in the units targeted for the survey who were eligible to participate and passively refused by not returning their survey or returning it blank without explicitly indicating their refusal to participate on the survey. In the absence of a returned survey with a marking on it to acknowledge the decision to participate (or not), we do not know whether the marine had the opportunity to participate in the survey.

Sociodemographic and Service History Characteristics

Respondents were asked to report their rank, age, ethnicity, race, marital status, number of children, military occupational specialty (MOS), and the number of previous deployments to Iraq or Afghanistan they had since 2001.[2]

Lifetime History of Potentially Traumatic Events

The Life Events Checklist (LEC) (Gray et al., 2004) was used to assess exposure to 17 different types of stressful events, such as a natural disaster, physical assault, assault with a weapon, combat or exposure to a war zone, life-threatening illness or injury, or serious injury, harm, or death the respondent caused to someone else. For each event, respondents indicated whether they had ever directly experienced the event, witnessed it, or learned about it. For each type of event assessed on the LEC, binary indicators were created to indicate whether the respondent had ever directly experienced the type of event or not (1 = had directly experienced the event, 0 = had not). In addition, a total score on the LEC was computed by summing the number of types of events that the respondent reported having directly experienced. Possible total scores on the LEC range from 0 to 17, where higher scores indicate that the respondent reported having directly experienced more types of potentially traumatic events in his or her lifetime.

Current Stress

Respondents were asked to rate their current level of stress on the COSC (e.g., green, yellow, orange, or red).

Lifetime History of PTSD Symptom Severity

Symptoms of PTSD were assessed with a modified version of the PTSD Checklist-Civilian Version (PCL-C) (Ruggiero et al., 2003). Respondents were asked to indicate on a five-point scale the extent to which they had experienced each of 17 symptoms "in your lifetime" as opposed to the standard time frame of the "past 30 days." A total scale score was computed by summing item responses. Possible scale scores range from 17 to 85, with higher scores indicating greater severity of PTSD symptoms experienced over the course of one's lifetime. This was used as a proxy for lifetime self-reported PTSD, for which no current self-report measure exists.

Depression

The Patient Health Questionnaire-2 (PHQ-2) (Kroenke, Spitzer, and Williams, 2003) was used to screen for MDD at baseline. This two-item screener assesses the frequency with which depressed mood and anhedonia, the inability to derive pleasure from activities once enjoyed, were experienced over the past two weeks on a 4-point (0–3) scale.

---

[2] Sex was not assessed on the survey due to concerns that this would greatly increase the risk of identifiability of female survey respondents, as females constitute a very small proportion of marines.

In our study, the time frame over which symptoms were assessed was the past month instead of the past two weeks.

High-Risk Alcohol Use

The AUDIT-C (Bush et al., 1998) was used to screen for high-risk alcohol use. This is a three-item measure that queries respondents about the frequency and quantity of their drinking over the past year. Possible scores range from zero to 12, and the higher the score, the more likely it is that the respondent's drinking is affecting his or her health and safety. Based on the U.S. Department of Veteran Affairs (VA)/DoD Clinical Practice Guideline for Management of Substance Use Disorders (The Management of Substance Use Disorders Working Group, 2009), which recommends a referral to specialty care for substance use disorders for individuals who have a score of eight or higher on the AUDIT-C, we used a cutoff score of eight or higher to categorize participants' self-reported drinking behavior as high risk. This cutoff score has been shown to have a sensitivity of .54 and a specificity of .94 in the detection of alcohol dependence in previous research (Dawson, 2005). Sensitivity refers to the proportion of individuals who have the condition (e.g., alcohol dependence) according to a gold-standard assessment, such as a structured clinical interview, and are correctly identified by the screener (e.g., AUDIT-C) as having the condition (e.g., 54 percent of individuals who met diagnostic criteria for alcohol dependence based on a structured clinical interview in a previous study by Dawson (2005) were correctly classified as having alcohol dependence using a cutoff score of eight or higher on the AUDIT-C. Specificity, in contrast, refers to the proportion of individuals who do not have the condition according to a gold-standard assessment and are correctly identified as not having the condition by the screener (e.g., 94 percent of individuals who did not meet criteria for alcohol dependence based on a structured clinical interview were correctly classified as not having alcohol dependence based on a score of less than eight on the AUDIT-C (Dawson, 2005).

Use of Social Resources for Stress and Potential Mental Health Problems

Respondents were asked about their use of different types of social resources in response to stress problems. Survey items assessed respondents' reports of both their own reliance on each of several resources for stress and their recommendation of the same resources to a "buddy" for help with stress. Possible resources included the following: oneself, buddy, leader, corpsman, chaplain, and unit medical officer.

Respondents were also asked how many times they had attended a stress class prior to or since joining their current unit and how often they had "taken action" when they or a buddy needed help with stress on a scale that ranged from "never" to "almost all of the time." Scores on these items were dichotomized to indicate whether the respondent reported having attended a stress class at least once in the past (1) versus never (0) and whether the respondent reported having taken action for stress most or all of the time (1) versus some of the time, rarely, or never (0).

Attitudes Toward Stress Response and Recovery

We assessed stress-related perceptions and attitudes, including respondents' self-perceived readiness; self-efficacy to handle their own stress and to help a peer handle his or her stress; the perceived efficacy of their peers and leaders to resolve their own stress problems and help the respondent resolve his or her stress problems; the extent to which they believe the responsibility to handle stress problems is shared by all marines; and the perceived stigmatization of or support for seeking help for stress problems at the level of the respondent's peers, leaders, unit, and the Marine Corps overall.

We developed two scales from these items: (1) positive expectancies toward coping with and recovering from stress and (2) perceived stigmatization of stress and seeking help for stress problems. Additional information is available in Appendix B. Possible and observed scores on both of the scales range from one to five. Higher scores connote more positive (i.e., healthier) perceptions and attitudes toward stress response and recovery.

Measure Properties

Additional information about these measures, including previous research on the psychometric properties of the survey measures and findings on the psychometric performance of the measures in the sample of pre-deployment survey participants, is available in Appendix B.

Statistical Analysis

Our primary goals in analyzing the pre-deployment survey were to

1. estimate the prevalence of stress and mental health problems in a sample of marines preparing for a combat deployment in support of OEF/OIF
2. examine the types and extent of resources used to cope with stress and mental health problems
3. identify service history characteristics (i.e., rank, type of battalion, and deployment history) that are associated with greater risk of experiencing stress and mental health problems, as well as with the differential use of resources for coping with stress and mental health problems.

We computed univariate descriptive statistics to accomplish the first two goals. We estimated bivariate associations between each of the service history characteristics and each of the outcomes of interest to accomplish the third goal.

Because scores on these variables were correlated within battalions, we adjusted for clustering at the level of the "parent" battalion in all univariate and bivariate analyses. We also created poststratification sampling weights so that the weighted sociodemographic and service history characteristics of our sample would approximate those of the target population the survey findings are intended to generalize: active-duty and reserve marines of rank O6 or lower who deployed to Iraq or Afghanistan sometime between March 2010 and December 2011. Sociodemographic and service history characteristics of the target population were determined from administrative data obtained from the Defense Manpower Data Center (DMDC).

All univariate and bivariate analyses were conducted in Stata to accommodate the sampling weights and clustering of observations within battalions. Rao-Scott chi-square tests were conducted to analyze bivariate associations between two categorical variables, and Wald tests were conducted to compare mean scores on continuous variables across groups (e.g., marines who had at least one previous deployment versus marines who had never previously deployed). Because we had three categories of rank (E1–E3, E4–E9, and officers), when analyzing differences by rank, we first conducted an omnibus significance test of differences between the three categories on the variable of interest. Then, only if the omnibus test was significant, we proceeded to conduct follow-up tests of significant differences between each pair of categories. In this way, we limited the number of significance tests to protect against the inflation of the Type 1 error rate.

CHAPTER FOUR

Results

In this chapter, we first describe the characteristics of the survey respondents and then present the results of our analysis in four areas: the estimated prevalence of mental health and stress conditions among marines prior to deployment; lifetime history of exposure to potentially traumatic events; the use of help-seeking resources and strategies for coping with stress; and attitudes toward stress response and recovery.

Survey Participants

To determine how closely our sample resembled the larger population of active-duty and reservist marines that our survey findings were intended to generalize, we obtained administrative data from DMDC on the entire population of marines of rank E1–E9 and O1–O6 who deployed to Iraq or Afghanistan during 2010 or 2011 and compared their sociodemographic and service history characteristics to those of our sample. Table 4.1 shows the sociodemographic and service history characteristics of OSCAR survey respondents and the larger population of marines the survey findings are intended to generalize.

Marines enrolled in the OSCAR evaluation were predominantly younger than age 25, white, junior enlisted (rank E1–E3), unmarried, and childless. Just over half of the marines in the sample had never deployed (i.e., they were preparing for their first deployment at the time of this survey), and just over half were in infantry as opposed to service support battalions. Compared to the larger population of marines, the sample of survey participants overrepresented marines who were under age 25, Hispanic, junior enlisted (E1–E3), unmarried, childless, and had previously deployed to Iraq or Afghanistan at least once since 2001.

Estimated Prevalence of Mental Health and Stress-Related Problems

The first phase of our analysis estimated the severity of PTSD symptoms experienced in one's lifetime; the prevalence of screening positive for current MDD, high-risk drink-

Table 4.1
Sociodemographic and Service History Characteristics of Marines Enrolled in the OSCAR Evaluation and of All Active-Duty and Reserve Marines

	Marines Enrolled in OSCAR Evaluation (N = 2,620)			All Marines[a] (N = 32,854)
Characteristic	**Unweighted Percentage**	**95% CI LL**	**95% CI UL**	**Percentage**
Age*				
At least 25 years old	21.1	16.3	25.9	39.1
Less than 25 years old	75.4	70.2	80.7	60.9
Race/ethnicity				
Hispanic*	18.1	13.6	22.6	13.0
Black or African American	6.3	4.2	8.4	7.9
White*	67.3	63.1	71.5	71.9
Asian*	2.0	1.5	2.5	3.2
Other	2.2	1.4	2.9	2.8
Rank				
E1–E3*	65.6	57.9	73.3	37.7
E4–E9*	25.9	19.4	32.3	48.5
Officer*	3.4	2.3	4.6	10.6
Married*	31.8	25.9	37.7	47.6
Has at least one child*	20.0	17.4	22.7	27.5
Number of previous deployments to Iraq or Afghanistan since 2001*				
0	55.8	46.5	65.2	74.8
1 or more	40.5	31.6	49.5	25.1
Battalion				
Infantry	57.5	21.2	93.7	N/A
Service support	42.5	6.3	78.8	N/A

SOURCE: Defense Manpower Data Center and study data.

NOTES: CI = Confidence Interval; LL = Lower Limit; UL = Upper Limit; N/A = Not Available; an asterisk indicates that the population value for all marines falls outside of the 95% CI around the corresponding point estimate for the sample of OSCAR marines, suggesting that the population value differs significantly from the point estimate for the sample of OSCAR marines.

[a] Active-duty and reserve marines of rank E1–E9 or O1–O6 who deployed to Iraq or Afghanistan in 2010 or 2011.

ing behavior, and stress problems, as well as the distributions of each type of problem by rank, battalion type, and deployment history.

The mean score on a modified version of the PCL that assessed the lifetime severity of PTSD symptoms was 32.0 (95% CI [30.8, 33.2]), where the possible range of scores was 17 to 85. Results from the PHQ-2 indicated that roughly one out of every eight marines (12.5%) screened positive for a probable diagnosis of MDD in the past 30 days.[1] Based on the AUDIT-C screening, 25.7 percent of respondents were identified as engaging in high-risk drinking. These results are displayed in Table 4.2.

About one-fifth of the sample (21.9%) reported that they or a buddy often needed help with stress. Although most participants were in the green (47.2%) or yellow (38.7%) stress continuum zone, a sizable minority (11.9%) reported that they were currently in the orange or red zone, suggesting difficulty coping with stress.

Table 4.2
Current Stress Level and Mental Health Burden (N = 2,620)

	Mean (95% CI)
Lifetime severity of PTSD symptoms[a]	32.0 (30.8, 33.2)
	Percentage (95% CI)
MDD probable diagnosis	12.5 (10.8, 14.2)
High-risk drinking	25.7 (22.7, 28.7)
Perceived need for help with stress for self or buddy (often or very often)	21.9 (16.3, 27.5)
Current stress continuum zone[b]	
Green (ready)	47.2 (41.5, 52.9)
Yellow (reacting)	38.7 (34.4, 43.0)
Orange (injured)	9.9 (6.5, 13.4)
Red (ill)	2.0 (0.8, 3.1)

NOTE: All estimates in the table are weighted to be representative of all marines of rank O6 or lower who deployed to Iraq or Afghanistan in 2010 or 2011.

[a] Lifetime severity of PTSD symptoms were assessed with a modified version of the 17-item PCL, in which respondents were asked to indicate the extent to which each symptom had been experienced "in your lifetime" instead of the standard time frame of "past 30 days." Each symptom was rated on a scale that ranged from 1 (not at all) to 5 (extremely). Composite scale scores range from 17 to 85.

[b] The percentages of respondents in different zones of the stress continuum sum to less than 100 percent due to missing data on this survey item (i.e., 2.2 percent of respondents declined to answer this survey question).

[1] It is important to note that the standard version of the PHQ-2 asks about depression symptoms over the past two weeks; in this study, symptoms were assessed over the past month. As a result, the estimate of probable MDD may be an overestimate.

To understand the characteristics that increase vulnerability to potential mental health and stress problems, we examined how the risk of self-reported mental health and stress problems is distributed across rank, type of battalion, and deployment history. Examining differences in mental health and stress burden by rank, we found that, in general, probable mental health and stress problems were more commonly reported by enlisted marines than by officers. Compared to officers, both groups of enlisted marines reported having experienced significantly greater PTSD symptom severity in their lifetimes, and a significantly higher proportion of junior enlisted marines (E1–E3) screened positive for probable MDD (see Table 4.3). High-risk drinking behavior was significantly more prevalent among junior enlisted marines relative to mid-level and senior enlisted marines, who in turn had higher rates of high-risk drinking behavior than officers.

A similar pattern was observed with respect to ratings of stress on the COSC: a significantly higher proportion of enlisted marines (13.4%) reported being in the orange or red zone than officers (0.8%). We did not observe significant differences in lifetime PTSD symptom severity, screening positive for depression, high-risk drinking, the frequency of perceived need for help with stress, or stress continuum ratings by battalion type (infantry versus service support) (see Appendix C, Table C.1).

Based on past research (Shen, Arkes, and Williams, 2012), we expected to find higher rates of mental health problems and higher levels of stress in marines who had previously deployed to Iraq or Afghanistan relative to those who had never deployed. Consistent with this expectation, we found that marines who had previously deployed to Iraq or Afghanistan reported significantly greater lifetime PTSD symptom severity relative to those who had never deployed (deployed once or more: M = 35.7, 95% CI [33.1, 38.2]; never deployed: M = 30.7, 95% CI [29.3, 32.1]). In addition, relative to marines who had never deployed, marines who had deployed at least once were more likely to report perceiving the need for help with stress for themselves or a buddy often or very often (deployed once or more: 27.8%; never deployed: 19.9%) and being in the orange or red zone of the COSC (deployed once or more: 15.4%; never deployed: 10.8%). However, those who had previously deployed did not differ from those who had never deployed in rates of probable current MDD or high-risk drinking. These comparisons are shown in Table 4.4.

Lifetime Rates of Potentially Traumatic Events

On average, marines in the sample reported that they had experienced approximately 4 (M = 3.9) types of potentially traumatic events over their lifetime out of a possible 17 types of events captured in the LEC. As illustrated in Table 4.5, the events most frequently reported were motor vehicle accidents (66.4%); the sudden, unexpected death of a loved one (45.4%); and physical assault (38.0%).

Table 4.3
Current Stress Level and Mental Health Burden, by Rank (N = 2,620)

	E1–E3 (n = 1,719)	E4–E9 (n = 725)	Officer (n = 90)
		Mean (95% CI)	
Lifetime severity of PTSD symptoms[a,b,d,e]	32.8 (31.3, 34.4)	32.7 (31.4, 34.0)	25.5 (22.2, 28.7)
		Percentage (95% CI)	
MDD probable diagnosis (current)[b,e]	15.3 (11.6, 19.0)	12.4 (10.6, 14.2)	3.3 (–2.7, 9.3)
High-risk drinking (current)[b,c,d,e]	33.1 (27.1, 39.0)	23.9 (20.8, 27.1)	7.5 (0.9, 14.1)
Perceived need for help with stress for self or buddy often or very often	23.4 (17.1, 29.7)	21.6 (15.6, 27.7)	17.6 (7.1, 28.1)
Current stress continuum zone[b,d,e,f]			
Green (ready)	46.4 (40.5, 52.3)	45.7 (39.0, 52.5)	57.3 (42.2, 72.3)
Yellow (reacting)	39.3 (34.4, 44.1)	37.9 (30.4, 45.4)	40.7 (26.1, 55.2)
Orange (injured)	9.3 (6.3, 12.3)	12.6 (7.1, 18.1)	0.1 (0, .13)
Red (ill)	2.6 (0.9, 4.3)	1.9 (0.1, 3.7)	0.03 (–0.03, 0.08)
	Enlisted		**Officer**
Orange or red (versus green or yellow)[b]	13.4 (9.7, 17.1)		0.08 (0, 0.16)

NOTE: All estimates in the table are weighted to be representative of all marines of rank O6 or lower who deployed to Iraq or Afghanistan in 2010 or 2011.

[a] Lifetime severity of PTSD symptoms were assessed with a modified version of the 17-item PCL in which respondents were asked to indicate the extent to which each symptom had been experienced "in your lifetime" instead of the standard time frame of "past 30 days." Each symptom was rated on a scale that ranged from 1 (not at all) to 5 (extremely). Composite scale scores range from 17 to 85.

[b] Rao-Scott chi-square test is statistically significant at $p < .05$.

[c] Difference between respondents of rank E1–E3 and rank E4–E9 is statistically significant at $p < .05$.

[d] Difference between respondents of rank E4–E9 and officers is statistically significant at $p < .05$.

[e] Difference between respondents of rank E1–E3 and officers is statistically significant at $p < .05$.

[f] Within columns, the percentages of respondents in different zones of the stress continuum sum to less than 100 percent due to missing data on this survey item.

When we assessed variation in reported history of potentially traumatic events by rank, we found that enlisted marines of rank E4–E9 reported experiencing significantly more types of potentially traumatic events on average (M = 4.3, 95% CI [3.8, 4.8]) than marines of rank E1–E3 (M = 3.5, 95% CI [3.3, 3.8]), who in turn reported

Table 4.4
Current Stress/Mental Health Burden, by Deployment History (N = 2,620)

	Never Deployed (n = 1,463)	Deployed Once or More (n = 1,062)
	Mean (95% CI)	
Lifetime severity of PTSD symptoms[a,b]	30.7 (29.3, 32.1)	35.7 (33.1, 38.2)
	Percentage (95% CI)	
MDD probable diagnosis (current)	12.4 (10.4, 14.4)	13.0 (9.3, 16.7)
High-risk drinking (current)	25.2 (21.8, 28.7)	27.1 (22.8, 31.4)
Perceived need for help with stress for self or buddy often or very often[b]	19.9 (13.1, 26.7)	27.8 (23.6, 32.1)
Current stress continuum zone[b,c]		
Green (ready)	47.2 (40.7, 53.8)	47.4 (41.9, 52.9)
Yellow (reacting)	39.6 (34.9, 44.2)	36.1 (31.7, 40.5)
Orange (injured)	8.9 (4.5, 13.4)	13.0 (11.2, 14.8)
Red (ill)	1.8 (0.5, 3.2)	2.4 (0.6, 4.2)
Orange or red (versus green or yellow)	10.8 (6.4, 15.1)	15.4 (13.2, 17.6)

NOTE: All estimates in the table are weighted to be representative of all marines of rank O6 or lower who deployed to Iraq or Afghanistan in 2010 or 2011.

[a] Lifetime severity of PTSD symptoms were assessed with a modified version of the 17-item PCL in which respondents were asked to indicate the extent to which each symptom had been experienced "in your lifetime" instead of the standard time frame of "past 30 days." Each symptom was rated on a scale that ranged from 1 (not at all) to 5 (extremely). Composite scale scores range from 17 to 85.

[b] Rao-Scott chi-square test is statistically significant at $p < .05$.

[c] Within columns, the percentages of respondents in different zones of the stress continuum sum to less than 100 percent due to missing data on this survey item.

experiencing significantly more types of potentially traumatic events than officers (M = 2.9, 95% CI [2.3, 3.5]) (see Appendix C, Table C.2). Relative to officers, significantly higher proportions of both E4–E9 marines and E1–E3 marines reported having experienced the sudden, unexpected death of a loved one; physical assault; exposure to a toxic substance; and a serious accident other than a motor vehicle accident. Marines of rank E4–E9 were also more likely than officers to report having experienced combat and having caused serious injury or death to another person.

We also found differences in lifetime history of potentially traumatic events by battalion type (see Appendix C, Table C.3). Marines in infantry battalions reported having experienced significantly more types of potentially traumatic events on average (M = 4.2, 95% CI [3.9, 4.5]) than marines in service support battalions (M = 3.6, 95% CI [3.3, 3.8]). In general, several types of events that may commonly occur in combat

Table 4.5
Lifetime History of Potentially Traumatic Events

	Marines (N = 2,620)	
Lifetime History of Traumatic Events	**Mean**	**95% CI**
Average number of potentially traumatic events directly experienced[a]	3.9	(3.6, 4.1)
Types of potentially traumatic events directly experienced	**Percentage**	**95% CI**
Motor vehicle accident	66.4	(62.6, 70.2)
Sudden, unexpected death of a loved one	45.4	(42.5, 48.4)
Other very stressful event	38.1	(35.0, 41.1)
Physical assault	38.0	(34.5, 41.5)
Other serious accident	29.0	(27.1, 31.0)
Natural disaster	28.2	(22.2, 34.2)
Fire/explosion	24.7	(21.8, 27.6)
Assault with a weapon	23.4	(19.9, 27.0)
Combat	19.2	(15.3, 23.2)
Caused the serious injury/death of another	13.6	(8.3, 19.0)
Exposure to toxic substance	14.8	(11.7, 18.0)
Witness violent death	10.6	(7.2, 14.1)
Life-threatening injury/illness	12.9	(11.2, 14.6)
Unwanted sexual experience other than sexual assault	6.3	(3.9, 8.8)
Severe human suffering	3.2	(1.8, 4.5)
Sexual assault	4.7	(2.6, 6.8)
Captivity	1.2	(0.7, 1.6)

NOTE: All estimates in the table are weighted to be representative of all marines of rank O6 or lower who deployed to Iraq or Afghanistan in 2010 or 2011.

[a] Participants were asked to indicate, for each of 17 traumatic events, whether they had directly experienced the event in their lifetime. The range of possible scores on this measure is 0 to 17.

(but not exclusively in combat) were more frequently endorsed by marines in infantry battalions relative to service support battalions, including combat itself, physical assault, assault with a weapon, having caused serious injury or death to another person, exposure to a toxic substance, witnessing a violent death, severe human suffering, and captivity.

There were, however, two types of events that were more commonly reported by marines in service support battalions than by marines in infantry battalions (also see Appendix C, Table C.3): sexual assault (service support: 6.5%, 95% CI [4.4, 8.5]; infantry: 2.7, 95% CI [0.9, 4.6]) and an unwanted sexual experience other than sexual assault (service support: 8.3%, 95% CI [4.5, 12.1]; infantry: 4.2%, 95% CI [3.0, 5.4]). It is not clear why marines in service support battalions would be more likely to report having experienced sexual assault or other unwanted sexual experiences; however, as sexual assault and other unwanted sexual experiences are more commonly reported by female service members than males, and at the time of this study females were in service support but not infantry battalions, differences in the gender composition of these two types of battalions may contribute to these findings. The absence of individual-level data on gender prevents us from examining whether these differences between service support and infantry battalions are attributable to gender differences. It is also possible that other differences between service support and infantry battalions, such as the mission focus, may contribute to the observed differences in rates of sexual assault and unwanted sexual experiences.

It might be expected that marines who had deployed at least once would have experienced more potentially traumatic events in their lifetime than those who had never deployed, given the greater exposure of the former group to combat during deployment. To evaluate this assumption, we compared the rate of occurrence of each type of potentially traumatic event and the average number of types of potentially traumatic events experienced among marines with and without a history of deployment. As shown in Table 4.6, the mean number of types of potentially traumatic events experienced was significantly higher among marines who had deployed at least once (M = 5.2, 95% CI [4.3, 6.1]) than among marines who had never deployed (M = 3.4, 95% CI [3.2, 3.5]). Similarly, marines who had previously deployed reported significantly higher rates of having experienced the sudden, unexpected death of a loved one; a serious accident other than a motor vehicle accident; combat; a fire or explosion; assault with a weapon; causing the serious injury or death of another; exposure to a toxic substance; witnessing a violent death; severe human suffering; and captivity. This is likely due to the increased chances of experiencing such traumatic events during a deployment.

Still, the proportion of marines who had never deployed that reported experiencing many types of traumatic events is notable. For example, 8 percent of those who had never deployed reported having caused serious injury or death to another; 22 percent had experienced assault with a weapon; and 44 percent had experienced the sudden, unexpected death of a loved one.

Use of Help-Seeking Resources for Stress

Most marines reported having attended a stress class at least once in the past (87.6%).

Table 4.6
Lifetime History of Potentially Traumatic Events, by Deployment History (N = 2,620)

	Never Deployed (n = 1,463)	Deployed Once or More (n = 1,062)
	Mean (95% CI)	
Average number of types of potentially traumatic events directly experienced[a,c]	3.4 (3.2, 3.5)	5.2 (4.3, 6.1)
Types of potentially traumatic events directly experienced[b]	Percentage (95% CI)	
Motor vehicle accident	65.1 (60.3, 70.0)	70.3 (65.6, 74.9)
Sudden, unexpected death of a loved one[c]	43.7 (40.2, 47.2)	50.7 (45.1, 56.3)
Other very stressful event[c]	35.2 (32.4, 38.1)	46.7 (39.2, 54.3)
Physical assault	37.4 (33.5, 41.3)	40.0 (35.0, 44.9)
Other serious accident[c]	27.9 (25.8, 30.1)	32.4 (27.9, 36.9)
Natural disaster	26.8 (21.3, 32.3)	32.5 (23.0, 42.0)
Combat[c]	3.3 (1.6, 5.0)	66.5 (54.4, 78.6)
Fire/explosion[c]	18.8 (15.6, 21.9)	42.5 (31.2, 53.8)
Assault with a weapon[c]	21.7 (18.6, 24.8)	28.5 (21.3, 35.7)
Caused serious injury/death of another[c]	8.2 (5.5, 10.9)	29.8 (16.2, 43.4)
Exposure to toxic substance[c]	11.7 (9.3, 14.0)	24.2 (16.2, 32.2)
Witness violent death[c]	6.0 (3.9, 8.2)	24.2 (14.4, 34.0)
Life-threatening injury/illness	12.6 (10.2, 15.0)	13.8 (8.9, 18.7)
Unwanted sexual experience other than sexual assault	6.9 (3.8, 10.1)	4.6 (2.2, 7.0)
Severe human suffering[c]	2.0 (1.00, 3.0)	6.6 (2.5, 10.7)
Sexual assault	5.0 (2.5, 7.5)	3.8 (1.7, 5.9)
Captivity[c]	0.9 (0.6, 1.2)	2.0 (0.6, 3.3)

NOTE: All estimates in the table are weighted to be representative of all marines of rank O6 or lower who deployed to Iraq or Afghanistan in 2010 or 2011.

[a] Participants were asked to indicate, for each of 17 traumatic events, whether they had directly experienced the event in their lifetime. The range of possible scores on this measure is 0 to 17. Cluster-adjusted Wald tests were conducted to determine whether there were significant differences by rank on the average number of potentially traumatic events experienced in one's lifetime.

[b] The Rao-Scott chi-square test was conducted to determine whether there were significant differences by rank in the percentage of respondents who reported having experienced each type of potentially traumatic event in their lifetime.

[c] There is a statistically significant difference between marines who had never deployed and those who had previously deployed at $p < .05$.

Table 4.7
Use of Help-Seeking Resources for Stress (N = 2,620)

	Percentage	(95% CI)
Stress class attended at least once since joining prior or current unit	87.6	(81.9, 93.3)
Used help-seeking resources for stress, by type		
Buddy	71.9	(68.5, 75.3)
Leader	49.7	(44.3, 55.0)
Corpsman	19.8	(16.8, 22.7)
Chaplain	21.0	(16.3, 25.8)
Unit medical officer	11.1	(9.2, 13.1)
Any	79.3	(74.8, 83.7)
Recommended help-seeking resources for stress, by type		
Buddy	84.0	(81.0, 86.9)
Leader	67.7	(62.9, 72.5)
Chaplain	60.5	(54.5, 66.6)
Corpsman	37.1	(32.5, 41.7)
Unit medical officer	28.3	(23.5, 33.2)
Any	88.7	(85.8, 91.5)

NOTE: All estimates in the table are weighted to be representative of all marines of rank O6 or lower who deployed to Iraq or Afghanistan in 2010 or 2011.

As shown in Table 4.7, most marines reported having used (79.3%) or recommended to a buddy (88.7%) one or more of the following resources for dealing with stress: a buddy, leader, chaplain, corpsman, or unit medical officer.

The most common type of resource used by respondents when dealing with their own stress was a buddy (71.9%). Similarly, the majority of marines reported having recommended a buddy as a resource when one of their buddies needed help with stress (84.0%). Leaders were the next most popular resource for help for oneself (49.7%) and to recommend to a buddy (67.7%).

Marines' reports of having used and/or recommended various types of resources for help with stress varied by rank, battalion, and deployment history. In general, marines of rank E4–E9 were more likely to report having used or recommended a resource for help dealing with stress (see Table 4.8). With regard to resources used to deal with one's own stress, marines of rank E4–E9 were significantly more likely than officers to report having used corpsmen (E4–E9: 20.7%; officers: 7.8%), chaplains (E4–E9: 23.7%; officers: 12.0%), and unit medical officers (E4–E9: 13.1%; officers:

Table 4.8
Percentage of Respondents Who Reported Help-Seeking Behaviors, by Rank (N = 2,620)

	Percentage (95% CI)		
	E1–E3 (n = 1,719)	E4–E9 (n = 725)	Officer (n = 90)
Used help-seeking resources for stress, by type			
Buddy	72.3 (68.7, 75.9)	69.0 (63.1, 74.9)	84.4 (74.5, 94.3)
Leader	48.1 (42.8, 53.4)	51.8 (42.1, 61.4)	46.3 (31.8, 60.7)
Corpsman[b,c,d]	21.9 (17.8, 25.9)	20.7 (16.5, 25.0)	7.8 (–0.1, 15.7)
Chaplain[b,d]	20.2 (14.6, 25.7)	23.7 (18.2, 29.1)	12.0 (2.2, 21.9)
Unit medical officer[b,d]	10.5 (7.7, 13.2)	13.1 (10.3, 15.8)	4.7 (–.4, 9.7)
Any	78.8 (75.2, 82.4)	78.0 (70.4, 85.7)	87.0 (77.8, 96.2)
Recommended help-seeking resources for stress, by type			
Buddy	81.7 (78.8, 84.6)	84.9 (80.8, 89.0)	88.3 (79.4, 97.2)
Leader	62.7 (58.0, 67.3)	70.9 (65.4, 76.4)	71.8 (55.7, 87.9)
Corpsman[a,b,c,d]	31.2 (25.9, 36.6)	44.9 (38.5, 51.2)	22.6 (14.4, 30.8)
Chaplain[a,c,d]	49.0 (40.8, 57.1)	68.5 (63.2, 73.7)	65.9 (55.5, 76.4)
Unit medical officer[a,d]	20.1 (15.2, 25.0)	35.0 (29.5, 40.6)	27.4 (16.7, 38.1)
Any	86.5 (84.2, 88.8)	90.3 (86.5, 94.2)	89.2 (79.9, 98.4)

NOTE: All estimates in the table are weighted to be representative of all marines of rank O6 or lower who deployed to Iraq or Afghanistan in 2010 or 2011.

[a] The difference between respondents of rank E1–E3 and rank E4–E9 is statistically significant at $p < .05$.

[b] The difference between respondents of rank E4–E9 and officers is statistically significant at $p < .05$.

[c] The difference between respondents of rank E1–E3 and officers is statistically significant at $p < .05$.

[d] Omnibus Rao-Scott chi-square test is statistically significant at $p < .05$.

4.7%). With respect to resources recommended to a buddy for help dealing with stress, marines of rank E4–E9 were significantly more likely than their lower-enlisted counterparts to report having recommended corpsmen (E4–E9: 44.9%; E1–E3: 31.2%), chaplains (E4–E9: 68.5%; E1–E3: 49.0%), and unit medical officers (E4–E9: 35.0%; E1–E3: 20.1%). Like their mid-level and senior enlisted peers, marines of rank E1–E3 were more likely than officers to report having used corpsmen to deal with their own stress (E1–E3: 21.9%; officers: 7.8%) and having recommended corpsmen to a buddy for help dealing with stress (E1–E3: 31.2%; officers: 22.6%). However, marines of rank

E1–E3 were significantly less likely than both marines of rank E4–E9 and officers to report having recommended a chaplain to a buddy for help with stress (E1–E3: 49.0%; E4–E9: 68.5%; officers: 65.9%).

We also observed significant variation by battalion type in the reported types of resources used for help with one's own stress and recommended to buddies for help with stress (see Appendix C, Table C.4). Specifically, marines in service support battalions were significantly more likely than their counterparts in infantry battalions to report having turned to buddies (service support: 73.8%; infantry: 69.9%), leaders (service support: 54.3%; infantry: 44.6%), and chaplains (service support: 25.3%; infantry: 16.2%) for help with their own stress and having recommended to a buddy the use of leaders for help with stress (service support: 71.1%; infantry: 64.0%). In contrast, marines in infantry battalions were significantly more likely than those in service support battalions to report having availed themselves of corpsmen for help dealing with their own stress (infantry: 23.8%; service support: 16.1%) and having recommended to a buddy the use of a corpsman for help with stress (infantry: 41.9%; service support: 32.7%). The latter findings are not surprising given that corpsmen are better represented, and therefore more accessible, in infantry battalions than in service support units.

We also found significant differences between marines who had previously deployed to Iraq or Afghanistan and marines who had never deployed in the types of resources recommended to a buddy for help with stress (see Appendix C, Table C.5). Marines who had previously deployed were significantly more likely than those who had never deployed to report having recommended any type of resource for help (ever-deployed: 91.0%; never-deployed: 88.0%), as well as each specific type of resource aside from a buddy: leaders (ever-deployed: 71.9%; never-deployed: 66.4%), corpsmen (ever-deployed: 44.5%; never-deployed: 34.6%), chaplains (ever-deployed: 70.9%; never-deployed: 57.1%), and unit medical officers (ever-deployed: 35.9%; never-deployed: 25.8%). There were no differences as a function of deployment history in the utilization of resources for help with one's own stress.

Attitudes Toward Stress Response and Recovery

We created two composite scales to measure (1) attitudes toward stress response and recovery and (2) perceived support for help-seeking among other marines. The individual items that constitute each scale were rated on a five-point Likert scale with response options that ranged from 1 (strongly disagree) to 5 (strongly agree) and were averaged to compute a composite scale score. Possible scores on these scales ranged from 1 to 5, with higher scores indicating more-positive, healthier attitudes. Additional detail regarding these scales can be found in Appendix B.

Attitudes Toward Stress Response and Recovery Scale

Generally, respondents reported positive attitudes toward stress response and recovery, agreeing with statements such as, "I can recognize signs of stress in my fellow marines" and "if I had a stress problem, I have buddies who would understand and help me get through it" (Table 4.9). The mean score on this scale was 4.01 (95% CI [3.97, 4.05]) out of a possible score of 5, where a higher score indicates a more positive attitude toward stress response and recovery. Table C.6 in Appendix C shows the item-by-item scoring results.

We found significant differences in attitudes toward stress response and recovery by rank (see Table 4.9 and Appendix C, Table C.7). Junior enlisted marines (E1–E3) reported the least positive attitudes toward stress response and recovery, with a mean score of 3.92 (95% CI [3.86, 3.97]), compared to E4–E9 marines (M = 4.06, 95% CI [4.00, 4.13]) and officers (M = 4.12, 95% CI [4.02, 4.22]). We also found a significant difference by deployment history (see Table 4.8 and Appendix C, Table C.8). Marines who had never deployed had significantly less positive attitudes toward stress response and recovery (M = 3.98, 95% CI [3.94, 4.03]) compared to marines who had deployed

Table 4.9
Attitudes Toward Stress Response and Recovery (N = 2,620)

	Mean Scale Score[a]	95% CI
Total sample	4.01	3.97, 4.05
By rank[b]		
E1–E3	3.92	3.86, 3.97
E4–E9	4.06	4.00, 4.13
Officer	4.12	4.02, 4.22
By deployment history[c]		
Never deployed	3.98	3.94, 4.03
Deployed at least once	4.10	4.04, 4.16
By battalion type		
Infantry	4.00	3.96, 4.05
Service support	4.02	3.96, 4.08

NOTE: All estimates in the table are weighted to be representative of all marines of rank O6 or lower who deployed to Iraq or Afghanistan in 2010 or 2011.

[a] Possible scores ranged from 1 to 5, with higher scores indicating more-positive, healthier attitudes.

[b] The difference between respondents of rank E1–E3 and rank E4–E9 and between respondents of rank E1–E3 and officers is statistically significant at $p < .05$.

[c] The difference between respondents who had never deployed and those who had deployed at least once is statistically significant at $p < .05$.

once or more (M = 4.10, 95% CI [4.04, 4.16]). We found no differences by battalion type (see Appendix C, Table C.9).

Perceived Support Scale

Respondents reported that they perceived moderate levels of support for help-seeking through some agreement with statements such as, "my leaders encourage seeking help for stress problems" and "the Marine Corps supports those who have mental health problems" (Table 4.10). The mean score on this scale was 3.12 (95% CI [3.06, 3.18]), where the range of possible scores is 1 to 5, and a higher score indicates greater perceived support for help-seeking. Appendix C, Table C.6, shows the item-by-item scoring results. We did not find any significant differences in perceived support for help-seeking by rank, deployment history, or battalion type (see Appendix C, Tables C.7, C.8, and C.9).

Comparison to Other Populations

We found that, even prior to their first deployment, marines in this study experienced a significant burden of mental health problems. We found high rates of positive screens for current MDD among marines who had never previously deployed. To place

Table 4.10
Perceived Support for Help-Seeking (N = 2,620)

	Mean Scale Score*	95% CI
Total sample	3.12	3.06, 3.18
By rank		
E1–E3	3.10	3.01, 3.19
E4–E9	3.12	3.04, 3.21
Officer	3.15	2.94, 3.36
By deployment history		
Never deployed	3.11	3.05, 3.17
Deployed at least once	3.14	3.05, 3.24
By battalion type		
Infantry	3.09	3.02, 3.17
Service support	3.14	3.07, 3.22

NOTE: All estimates in the table are weighted to be representative of all marines of rank O6 or lower who deployed to Iraq or Afghanistan in 2010 or 2011.

* Possible scores ranged from 1 to 5, with higher scores indicating more-positive, healthier attitudes.

these findings in context, we compared them to estimates of the prevalence of current depression among adult males in the U.S. general population based on a nationally representative dataset, the Behavioral Risk Factor Surveillance System (BRFSS) (see Table 4.11).

In the BRFSS, the rate of current depression among adult males in the U.S. general population was 6.4 percent (Kroenke et al., 2009) compared to 12.4 percent of marines in our study who had never deployed and screened positive for current MDD. However, it is important to note that the BRFSS employed a different measure of depression than that used in our study,[2] and that the age distribution of BRFSS participants differs from that of the marines in the current study, which could partially account for the observed discrepancies in rates of depression.

Another nationally representative survey, the 2001–2002 National Epidemiological Survey on Alcohol and Related Conditions (NESARC), which used a measure of alcohol misuse, is nearly identical to the one we employ.[3] According to the NESARC, 16.1 percent of adult males in the U.S. general population of similar age to the OSCAR survey respondents reported high-risk drinking behavior, as measured by the same

Table 4.11
Mental Health Burden Among Marines Versus National Estimates

	Percentage of Marines Enrolled in OSCAR Evaluation (n = 2,620)	Percentage of Marines Enrolled in OSCAR Evaluation Never Deployed (n = 1,463)	Percentage of Marines Enrolled in OSCAR Evaluation Who Had Deployed Once or More (n = 1,062)	Estimated Percentage of U.S. General Population
MDD probable diagnosis (current)	12.5	12.4	13.0	6.4
High-risk drinking (current)	25.7	25.2	27.1	16.1

NOTE: All estimates in the table are weighted to be representative of all marines of rank O6 or lower who deployed to Iraq or Afghanistan in 2010 or 2011.

SOURCES: Behavioral Risk Factor Surveillance System (Kroenke et al., 2009); National Epidemiological Survey on Alcohol and Related Conditions; RAND analysis.

---

[2] The BRFSS employed the Patient Health Questionnaire-8 (Kroenke, Spitzer, and Williams, 2001; Löwe et al., 2004) to assess depression, whereas our study employed the PHQ-2, which is comprised of the first two items of the PHQ-8. Unfortunately, there are no nationally representative data available on the percentage of adults in the U.S. general population who screen positive for depression on the PHQ-2.

[3] The NESARC used a derived version of the AUDIT-C that corresponds very closely to the original version of the AUDIT-C with the primary difference pertaining to an item on the frequency of binge drinking. In the NESARC, respondents are asked how often they drink "5 or more drinks in a single day," as opposed to "6 or more drinks on one occasion" as in the original AUDIT-C.

AUDIT-C cutoff applied in our study.[4] In comparison, 25.2 percent of marines who had never deployed reported high-risk drinking.

We also found that lifetime rates of reported exposure to potentially traumatic events were higher than expected, even among marines who had never previously deployed to Iraq or Afghanistan. To put our findings in context, we compared them to findings from the National Comorbidity Survey (NCS), a nationally representative survey in which respondents were asked to indicate which of several types of potentially traumatic events they had directly experienced in their lifetime (Kessler et al., 1995). In comparison to adult males in the U.S. general population, a higher proportion of marines who had never deployed reported having experienced different types of potentially traumatic events (see Table 4.12). Over one-third (37.4%) of marines who had never deployed reported having directly experienced physical assault compared with 11.1 percent of males in the U.S. general population. Just over one-quarter (26.8%) of marines who had never deployed reported having experienced a natural disaster compared with 18.9 percent of the U.S. general male population, and 5.0 percent of marines who had never deployed reported having experienced a sexual assault compared with 0.7 percent of males in the U.S. general population.

Table 4.12
Percentages of OSCAR Marines Who Experienced Different Types of Potentially Traumatic Events in Their Lifetime Compared with National Estimates

Traumatic Event	All OSCAR Marines (n = 2,620)	Never Deployed (n = 1,463)	Deployed Once or More (n = 1,062)	U.S. General Population Estimate
Physical assault	38.0	37.4	40.0	11.1
Natural disaster	28.2	26.8	32.5	18.9
Sexual assault	4.7	5.0	3.8	0.7

NOTE: All estimates in the table are weighted to be representative of all marines of rank O6 or lower who deployed to Iraq or Afghanistan in 2010 or 2011.

[4] The rate of high-risk drinking behavior (16.1%) among adult males in the U.S. general population with the same age distribution as that of the OSCAR survey respondents was computed directly from the NESARC dataset for the purpose of comparison with the findings reported in this study.

CHAPTER FIVE

Conclusions and Recommendations

The results of this survey provide both a baseline picture to permit assessment of the effects of the OSCAR program, as well as an understanding of the overall mental health needs of marines, which is necessary for ensuring that adequate resources are available to support this population. Other RAND research has found that DoD lacks a needs assessment that addresses psychological health among the populations targeted by its programs (Weinick et al., 2011). Our findings help address that gap by identifying the magnitude of observed pre-deployment mental health challenges among marines. In this chapter, we summarize key findings and provide recommendations for addressing the pre-deployment psychological health needs of marines.

Marines Have Significant Pre-Deployment Mental Health Burdens

Marines in this study had high pre-deployment mental health needs relative to the general population.

- The rates of current probable diagnosis of MDD were higher among marines than among the general population, even for those marines who had never deployed.[1]
- Marines were also more likely than their counterparts in the general U.S. population to have been exposed to traumatic events. In general, for types of traumatic events other than those that are more likely to occur in the context of a combat-related deployment,[2] there was no difference in rates of exposure between marines who had never deployed and those who had deployed at least once.

[1] As noted in the preceding chapter, the nationally representative study of the U.S. general population that served as the standard to which the marines in the current study were compared on current probable diagnosis of MDD used a different measure of depression than that used in the current study, and the sample had a different age distribution (i.e., a greater range and greater variability, consistent with the U.S. general population) than that of the sample of marines in the current study. These differences in measurement and sample composition could help to explain the observed differences between males in the U.S. general population and marines in the current study in rates of current probable diagnosis of MDD.

[2] Types of traumatic events that are more likely to occur in the context of a combat-related deployment for which there were significant differences by history of deployment were sudden, unexpected death of a loved one; serious accident other than motor vehicle accident; combat; fire or explosion; assault with a weapon; causing the

- Marines are more likely to report engaging in high-risk drinking than their counterparts in the general U.S. population; rates are equally high among those marines who have never deployed and those who have deployed at least once.

Recommendation 1. Consider implementing programs to identify and address mental health issues, such as PTSD, MDD, lifetime history of traumatic events, and high-risk drinking prior to deployment.

There are numerous programs to support the post-deployment mental health needs of marines (Weinick et al., 2011); however, there are few that identify and address the mental health burden of marines prior to a deployment. Current DoD policy and a congressional mandate require that all service members receive a pre-deployment mental health screening (HR 2647, 2009). This screening is intended to be conducted hand-in-hand with routine physical health screenings to determine which service members are mentally fit for deployment. There is evidence from the Army that such screening is effective at reducing the prevalence of mental health problems in theater when it is combined with coordinated in-theater treatment of those with existing mental health problems (Warner et al., 2011b). However, such a strategy has not been tested for marines.

Understanding the preexisting mental health burden of a unit before deployment could help leaders to better anticipate the mental health problems and needs of their marines during and after a deployment. Programs like OSCAR could be augmented to include information about the impact of preexisting (i.e., pre-deployment) mental health burdens and stressors. Programs in which embedded mental health providers (Greden et al., 2010) have advance knowledge of mental health problems and can identify marines who should be seen regularly during and after a deployment may also be helpful, though research into the potential benefits and consequences of such an approach is warranted.

However, since the required screening is conducted "on the record," marines may not accurately report their symptoms for fear of being disqualified from deployment or experiencing other career harms. A screening program developed and administered by a third party, as well as treatment services available outside the military health system, may be helpful in addressing this concern.

Recommendation 2. Investigate the relationship between pre-deployment mental health burden, experiences while in theater, and the likelihood of developing longer-term mental health problems.

While our data reveal significant levels of potential mental health problems prior to deployment, little is known about the relationship between pre-deployment mental

---

serious injury or death of another; exposure to a toxic substance; witnessing a violent death; severe human suffering; and captivity.

health, combat experiences, and longer-term mental health. In addition, little is known about factors, such as personality traits, that influence individuals' resilience and response to traumatic events. Further study in these areas could help in developing models that better identify marines who are at risk for exacerbated mental health problems during or after deployment and allow for the provision of services designed to prevent such longer-term problems.

Junior Enlisted Marines May Be More At-Risk Than Others

This study showed that probable mental health problems are three to four times more prevalent among enlisted marines compared to officers, and that junior enlisted marines (rank E1–E3) had the highest rates of probable mental health problems. In particular, a third (33%) of junior enlisted marines have high-risk alcohol use compared to 24 percent of more highly ranked enlisted marines (rank E4–E9) and 8 percent of officers. The prevalence of high-risk drinking among junior enlisted marines is twice as high as in a civilian population sample of similarly aged males.[3]

In addition, junior enlisted marines are less likely than marines of higher ranks to have a positive attitude toward combat and operational stress and the ability of a marine to recover from stress problems. For example, junior enlisted marines assigned lower scores to statements such as, "it's possible to recover from a stress injury or illness and do your job as well as before" and were less likely than more highly ranked marines to endorse statements such as, "members of my unit would have more confidence in me if I sought help for a stress problem" (see Appendix C, Table C.8).

Recommendation 3. Target prevention and treatment efforts to junior enlisted marines.

Such targeted services could help in supporting those marines who are most likely to experience mental health challenges prior to deployment. Efforts targeted toward drinking behaviors may be especially important given the elevated rates of high-risk drinking among junior enlisted marines.

Recommendation 4. Consider additional training on combat and operational stress for junior enlisted marines.

While the OSCAR program is designed to provide training in combat and operational stress control to battalion leaders, the findings from this survey suggest that junior enlisted marines could also benefit from education about stress, as well as an increased understanding of the resources available within the Marine Corps.

---

[3] Based on RAND's analysis of NESARC data. See Chapter Four.

Marines Have Generally Positive Attitudes Toward Stress and Use Available Help-Seeking Resources

The marines in our sample generally expressed positive attitudes toward stress response and recovery, and they perceived moderate levels of support for seeking help related to mental health problems. However, some stigma around mental health problems was evidenced by moderate agreement with statements such as, "if I sought help to deal with stress, my unit leadership might treat me differently" and "I would be seen as weak if others knew I needed help with stress" (see Appendix C, Table C.6).

Most marines reported having previously attended a class for stress and having used or recommended to a buddy one of several common resources, including a buddy, leader, chaplain, or medical personnel.

Recommendation 5. Continue efforts to reduce the stigma around mental health problems and help-seeking in the Marine Corps.

While the findings from our survey suggest that most marines have positive attitudes about combat and operational stress and confidence in their ability to react to stress, the findings also suggest some stigma around receiving help for stress or mental health problems. Programs such as OSCAR may be well positioned to help reduce the stigma associated with mental health problems. A preliminary assessment of the effects of another military program called Buddy-to-Buddy, which also uses peers to reduce the stigma of seeking help among returning soldiers in the Michigan Army National Guard, provides tentative support for the notion that peer support programs can be successful at reducing stigma (Greden et al., 2010). To effectively do so, it may be helpful for training messages to focus on mental health problems as part of a range of reactions to combat and operational stress and to emphasize help-seeking as an appropriate response.

Recommendation 6. Continue to make multiple resources for help available to accommodate varied preferences.

Marines reported using a wide variety of resources when in need of help for stress. The types of resources used and recommended to buddies were found to vary by rank, battalion type, and deployment history. Of particular interest, junior-enlisted marines were more likely than officers to recommend corpsmen to buddies as a resource for coping with stress, but less likely than officers to recommend chaplains. In addition, those in service support units were more likely to rely on chaplains, while those in infantry units more commonly relied on corpsmen. Routinely training a range of individuals to identify the warning signs of mental health problems, support marines in times of stress, and refer them to care when needed can help ensure that the preferred resources are available for all marines in times of need.

Further, to encourage marines to seek care when needed, it must be clear to them that the career repercussions associated with seeking help are limited and that receiving such help when needed is supported by Marine Corps leadership.

Limitations of This Study

While the findings of this study are important, there are several limitations to our methods that should be noted. First, our sample is a convenience sample rather than a random sample. We did develop sampling weights so that our sample would better represent the population of marines who deployed to Iraq or Afghanistan during the same time frame as the marines who participated in our study. Still, it is possible that there is some unmeasured characteristic on which our sample differs from the population, so the estimates of mental health and stress problems produced here may not closely resemble the true population values. Second, the measure of depression used here is a screener, which is not intended to yield actual diagnoses of current MDD. If full diagnostic interviews were conducted, it is likely that the prevalence of diagnosed MDD would be lower. Additionally, we chose to assess lifetime history of PTSD symptoms rather than measure current PTSD symptoms. However, we were unable to determine lifetime history of PTSD diagnoses. A diagnosis of PTSD can be made only in the context of a formal diagnostic interview, which was not possible in this study.

Concluding Observation

Because most analyses of the mental health and well-being of military service members have focused on post-deployment issues, so too have most DoD programs for addressing stress-related problems arising from deployment. However, our results indicate the presence of a substantial pre-deployment mental health burden in the sample of marines we surveyed. This suggests that pre-deployment mental health concerns deserve greater attention within the Marine Corps and potentially throughout DoD, and that additional research is called for to understand service members' mental health burden across the full deployment cycle and how those with mental health problems can best be supported.

APPENDIX A

Description of the OSCAR Program and RAND's Evaluation

Description of the OSCAR Program

The OSCAR program includes several components that were developed and implemented in phases between 2006 and 2012. The data described in this report were collected between March 2010 and December 2011. At that time, the OSCAR program conducted three main activities: (1) embedding mental health providers in Marine Corps regiments, (2) training other medical personnel to address combat and operational stress control problems, and (3) training selected officers and senior NCOs to act as first responders for marines with stress injuries. In conducting these activities, the OSCAR program made use of four types of individuals:

1. *OSCAR Providers*—mental health providers embedded in Marine Corps regiments. These providers deploy with the regiment and are available in theater to support the mental health needs of marines.
2. *OSCAR Extenders*—selected physicians, dental officers, nurses, other medical service providers, chaplains, religious program specialists, and senior corpsmen. These individuals receive specific training in supporting marines who experience combat and operational stress problems.
3. *OSCAR Team Members*—officers and senior NCOs. OSCAR team members attend a one-day (6–8 hours) training course conducted by OSCAR master trainers. Relative to OSCAR providers and extenders, OSCAR team members are closer to the field and the small-unit level, giving them the earliest opportunity to identify and support marines in distress. The support they provide includes assistance with the mitigation of controllable stressors, psychological first aid for marines experiencing acute stress reactions, referrals to OSCAR extenders and/or providers (e.g., chaplains, corpsmen, mental health professionals) for help with more severe stress problems, and the facilitation of an individual's reintegration into the unit following treatment for severe stress problems.
4. *OSCAR Master Trainers*—marines who have successfully completed a train-the-trainer course and are authorized to conduct OSCAR team member training.

Our evaluation of OSCAR focuses exclusively on the OSCAR team member component, as this is the most well-defined and widely implemented component of the program. Below we describe the theoretical framework of the OSCAR team member training and provide additional details about the expected role of OSCAR team members.

OSCAR Team Member Training

Trained personnel conduct OSCAR team member training using an interactive group presentation format. Commanding officers select officers and NCOs from their unit to attend the training on the basis of their perceived ability to lead effectively, serve as a positive role model, and help and mentor marines with stress problems. The group sessions include an overview of the OSCAR program objectives, information on the biological basis of stress reactions and their social/behavioral impacts on soldiers, implications for mission readiness among soldiers and units, and the ways in which the OSCAR program seeks to improve the management of combat stress. The trainers also lead group discussions and conduct role-playing exercises designed to help the officers and NCOs practice the skill sets important for preventing, identifying, and managing stress problems among marines. The training concludes with a panel of experienced marines who share their own experiences with combat stress and discuss how the principles of the OSCAR program apply to them. Typically, the OSCAR training is delivered during a single day and lasts from morning until mid-afternoon.

OSCAR team member training is conducted as part of a battalion's deployment preparations. Typically, OSCAR training occurs three to five months before the battalion deploys. OSCAR team members are expected to employ the skills they gained in the training both during and after a deployment, though the biggest impact of the training on a particular battalion is likely to be felt during deployment. The most recent set of OSCAR training guidelines distributed by the Marine Corps Combat Operational Stress Control office in October 2011 mandated that all battalions in the Marine Corps assemble and train an OSCAR team by January 31, 2012. These guidelines require that each battalion's OSCAR team consist of a minimum of five percent of the battalion's personnel or 20 marines and sailors, whichever is greater. The OSCAR team members (i.e., small-unit leaders who attend OSCAR training) (Nash and Watson, 2012) constitute the majority of the OSCAR team.

The OSCAR team member training is based on the COSC model. This model describes responses to combat and operational stress along a spectrum of possible outcomes that range in severity from "adaptive coping" and "full readiness" to clinical mental disorders. The COSC model (see Figure A.1) applies four possible categories to its continuum, which are color-coded as green ("ready"), yellow ("reacting"), orange ("injured"), and red ("ill").

Figure A.1
Marine Corps Combat and Operational Stress Continuum

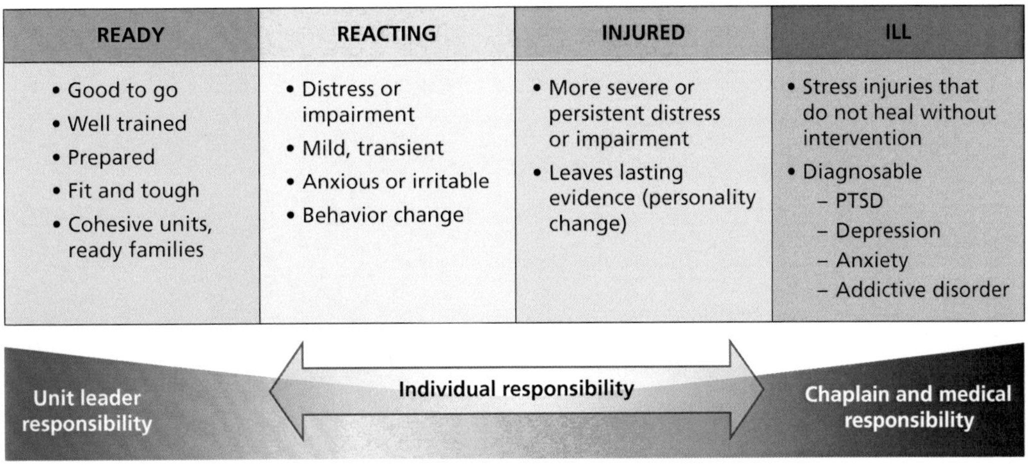

READY	REACTING	INJURED	ILL
• Good to go • Well trained • Prepared • Fit and tough • Cohesive units, ready families	• Distress or impairment • Mild, transient • Anxious or irritable • Behavior change	• More severe or persistent distress or impairment • Leaves lasting evidence (personality change)	• Stress injuries that do not heal without intervention • Diagnosable – PTSD – Depression – Anxiety – Addictive disorder

Unit leader responsibility
Individual responsibility
Chaplain and medical responsibility

SOURCE: U.S. Marine Corps, 2010.
RAND *RR218-A.1*

The Role of OSCAR Team Members

Building on the COSC model, the Navy and Marine Corps identified five "core leader functions" to promote psychological health and build resilience (see Figure A.2). All Navy and Marine Corps leaders, including the officers and senior NCOs who receive training to become an OSCAR team member, should (1) *strengthen* their marines and sailors by fostering unit cohesion and exposing them to realistic training, (2) *mitigate* stress by ensuring their marines get adequate rest and by removing unnecessary stressors, (3) *identify* signs of stress in their marines and sailors, (4) *treat* stress with rest and restoration or referral to a chaplain or mental health provider, and (5) *reintegrate* marines and sailors who have recovered from a stress problem back into the unit.

OSCAR team members are intended to be "first responders" for marines experiencing combat and operational stress. Relative to OSCAR providers and extenders, OSCAR team members are closer to the field and the small-unit level, giving them the earliest opportunity to identify a marine in distress. The primary role of OSCAR team members is to conduct the core leader functions described above to prevent marines from entering into the orange (injured) or red (ill) zones of the COSC. These actions are further specified below:

- *Strengthen*: OSCAR team members should help expand their marines' capacity for stress so that they can withstand greater amounts of stress and still remain in the green and yellow zones.
- *Mitigate*: OSCAR team members should pay attention to different sources of stress affecting their marines, including not only combat-related problems but

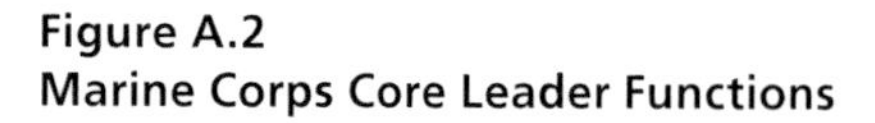

Figure A.2
Marine Corps Core Leader Functions

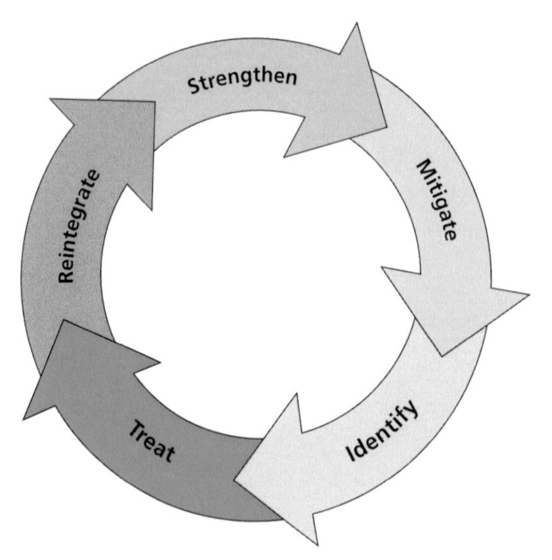

SOURCE: U.S. Marine Corps, 2010.
RAND *RR218-A.2*

other concerns such as finances, relationship problems, health problems, or other issues. The goal for leaders is to recognize possible problems early and help their marines keep their overall stress levels manageable, partly by mitigating more-controllable stressors (e.g., conflicts with superiors) to conserve coping resources for less-controllable stressors (e.g., seeing a buddy injured in combat). Leaders can also mitigate stress problems by reducing the stigma of stress problems within the unit and demonstrating that it is possible to learn from stressful experiences through posttraumatic growth. OSCAR team members can do this by talking openly to the marines in their unit about such issues (e.g., sharing their own experiences with stress, including healthy stress management approaches and their positive outcomes); conveying an attitude of acceptance and encouragement to marines in their unit who are receiving help for stress problems; and generally modeling healthy attitudes and behaviors toward stress management.

- *Identify*: Leaders are expected to "know their marines" (i.e., be familiar with the typical mood, behavior, appearance, and body language of each of their marines) so that they can detect changes that may indicate a burgeoning stress problem. Following a mission, leaders are encouraged to use the After Action Review, in which the unit members review the strengths and weaknesses of their performance, as an opportunity to look for behavioral changes in their marines.
- *Treat*: If an OSCAR team member notices signs indicating that a marine is in the yellow, orange, or red zone of the COSC, he or she is advised to take action, with the stipulation that "treating" is not meant to imply that unit leaders should act as

clinicians but rather intervene early with a marine exhibiting stress problems and help ensure they get into clinical care. OSCAR team members can intervene by
- ensuring physical needs are met (e.g., providing a period of rest)
- providing psychological first aid, which includes engaging with the marine, providing safety and comfort, gathering information and providing practical assistance, and connecting the marine with social support and information on coping (Nash and Watson, 2012)
- referring those with urgent need for medical attention to a mental health professional and facilitating mental health treatment adherence.

- *Reintegrate*: OSCAR team members should mentor marines who have experienced stress problems (and received mental health treatment) to prepare them to return to duty. An important element of reintegration is reducing the stigma related to seeking treatment.

Evaluation of the OSCAR Program

To understand whether the OSCAR program, in particular the OSCAR team member component, is meeting its objectives, our research team gathered survey data from marines and OSCAR team members and conducted qualitative discussions with marines and battalion leaders.

Specifically, the evaluation approach included:

- longitudinal surveys of marines from OSCAR-trained and non–OSCAR-trained battalions designed to assess the impact of OSCAR on mission readiness, unit cohesion, mental health stigma, and stress burden
- longitudinal surveys of OSCAR team members designed to assess team member perceptions of the OSCAR program and its effect on mission readiness and force preservation
- semistructured interviews with commanding officers of battalions that had received OSCAR training
- focus groups with battalion leaders, health care providers, and chaplains who had received OSCAR training prior to deployment.

The longitudinal surveys of marines and OSCAR team members were conducted at two different times. The first survey was conducted pre-deployment, before a battalion received OSCAR team member training. The second survey was conducted within two months of redeployment.

Detailed information about the overall evaluation and complete findings will be available in a future report.

APPENDIX B

Additional Methodological Detail

Sampling

Three of the battalions sampled were augmented by marines from other battalions prior to deployment to form larger composite units, each of which functioned as a single unit during deployment. All of these were service support battalions, such as combat logistics or engineering support battalions. Collectively, these three composite battalions included marines from ten "parent" battalions. The three composite service support battalions ranged in size from 222 marines to 452 marines, with an average (mean) of 371 marines (SD = 129) in each battalion. The ten "parent" battalions ranged in size from 10 marines to 349 marines, with an average (mean) of 111 marines (SD = 129) in each battalion. The other four battalions sampled, all infantry, were not augmented by other battalions. The size of the four infantry battalions ranged from 322 marines to 514 marines, with an average (mean) of 377 marines (SD = 92) in each battalion. Altogether, the seven battalions (the three composite service support battalions and four infantry battalions) included marines from 14 "parent" battalions. Of the seven battalions, all four infantry battalions and one of the service support battalions received OSCAR training after the pre-deployment survey and prior to deployment; the remaining two service support battalions did not receive OSCAR training prior to deployment.

We sampled between three and five companies from each of the four infantry battalions. For the first two infantry battalions, companies were randomly sampled within the battalion. Because random sampling proved very logistically challenging to implement, we sampled all available companies from the two remaining infantry battalions.

For two of the composite service support battalions, we also attempted to recruit all available companies in the battalion. From the third composite service support battalion, we sampled only two companies (one from the main battalion, one from another battalion that was augmenting the main battalion) because this recruitment fully met our targeted sample size.

Figure B.1 depicts the sampling strategy.

Figure B.1
Sampling Strategy

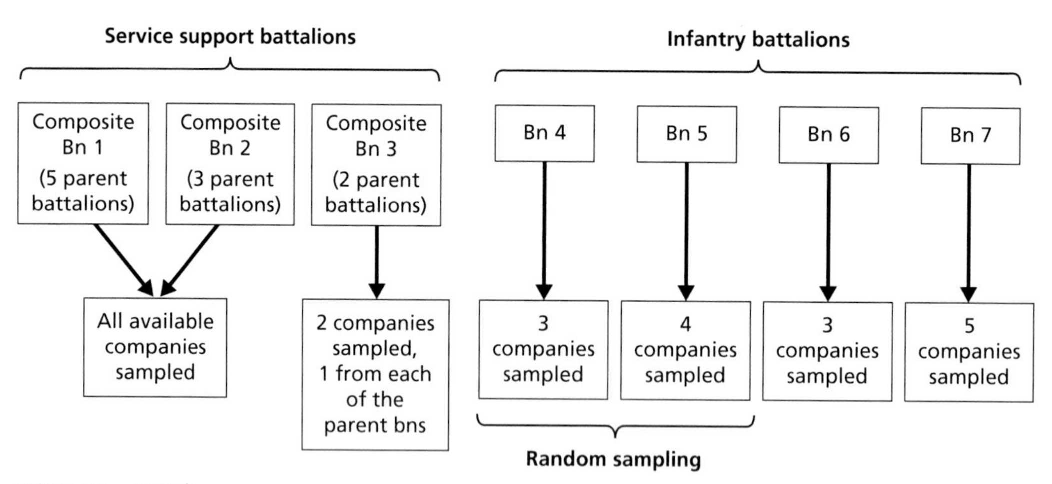

NOTE: Bn = Battalion.
RAND *RR218-B.1*

Procedures

Once a subset of companies to target for recruitment had been identified within each battalion, we coordinated with a point of contact (POC) in the unit to determine a date and time when the majority of the marines would be available to take the survey. The unit POC then arranged for the marines to come to the survey administration site at the agreed-upon date and time. Before the survey was administered, a survey administrator would read the Human Subjects Protection Committee (HSPC)–approved oral consent script describing the study's purpose and relevant information about human subjects' research protections (e.g., the voluntary nature of participation, protection of the confidentiality of survey responses). After this script was read, the marines were asked to decide whether to participate and to indicate their decision on the front page of the survey. All marines, regardless of whether they chose to participate, were asked to return their survey to the survey administrator in the blank envelope provided with the survey after they were finished.

Given that military populations are accustomed to following orders and the potential for prospective survey participants to misconstrue the survey as mandatory, several measures were taken to avert this misperception and mitigate pressure to participate in the study. Survey arrangements were coordinated with a unit POC who was not in the chain of command—typically a marine in the operations section (S-3). Unit commands were not permitted to be in the room at the time of survey administration. Survey administrators were required to be outside of the chain of command and typically included members of the RAND team, COSC personnel, or the unit chaplain or religious program specialist. Prior to administering the survey, administrators who were not RAND staff were required to read survey administration instructions that delineated their role in protecting the confidentiality of individual marines' decisions regarding participation and survey responses, and they were required to affirm in writing (or via email) their understanding and agreement to abide by the prescribed survey procedures.

We also took care to communicate to prospective participants the nature and extent of the protections applied to maintain the confidentiality of individual survey responses and the purpose for which survey data were being collected. Similar questionnaires that cover sensitive topics such as mental health and alcohol use (e.g., PDHA), are routinely used in the military to inform decisions regarding the screening, referral, and treatment of mental health and substance use problems and are included in the individual's military record. To distinguish our survey from these similar questionnaires used in the military, we emphasized in the oral consent script and survey instructions that the participant's individual responses to this survey would be used only for research, would never be shared with anyone outside of the RAND research team, and would never be tied to their military record in any way. This clarification was important both from a human subjects' protections standpoint and from a data quality standpoint, given the research indicating that mental health problems tend to be underestimated when based on data collected without anonymity, as in the PDHA (Warner et al., 2011a).

Measures Drawn from Existing Instruments

Life Events Checklist

The LEC is designed to assess a respondent's lifetime history of potentially traumatic events. Past research has documented the adequacy of the LEC's temporal stability and convergent validity with another established measure of trauma exposure (Gray et al., 2004). Importantly, the convergent validity of the LEC has also been demonstrated in a sample of combat veterans via its associations with measures of psychological distress and PTSD symptoms (Gray et al., 2004).

PTSD Checklist—Civilian Version

The original PCL was developed by Weathers et al. (1993) and is designed to measure symptoms of PTSD. It contains 17 symptom items keyed directly to the *Diagnostic and Statistical Manual of Mental Disorder,* 4th Edition (American Psychiatric Association, 1994). Respondents are asked to rate each of the items on a five-point scale according to how much the symptom has "bothered" them in the past 30 days, with higher ratings indicating greater symptom severity. In our study, a slightly modified version of the PCL was used, in which respondents were asked to indicate the extent to which they had experienced each of the 17 symptoms "in your lifetime" as opposed to the "past 30 days." A composite scale score was computed by summing the item responses. Possible scale scores range from 17 to 85, with higher scores indicating greater severity of PTSD symptoms experienced over the course of one's lifetime. Internal consistency reliability for this measure in our study was excellent (Cronbach's alpha = 0.95).

Patient Health Questionnaire-2

The PHQ-2 is a brief measure of mental health that has been validated as a measure of depression against an independent, structured mental health professional interview in past research (Kroenke et al., 2009). A cutoff score of three or greater on the PHQ-2 has been shown to have a sensitivity of 83 percent and a specificity of 92 percent for detecting MDD (Kroenke, Spitzer, and Williams, 2003). However, it is important to note that the standard reference time frame for the PHQ-2 is "in the past two weeks," and in our study the reference time frame was "in the past month." It is not known to what extent this changes the sensitivity and specificity of the measure for detecting MDD.

AUDIT-C

The AUDIT-C has been validated as a screener for the identification of individuals with heavy drinking and/or active alcohol abuse or dependence in the past (Bush et al., 1998; Dawson, 2005). This self-report measure includes three items that assess the quantity and frequency of typical and heavy drinking. In our study, frequency of drinking behavior was assessed without respect to a specific time frame in the past, and quantity of drinking behavior was assessed with respect to "a typical day when you are drinking." Participants answer each item on a 0–4 scale, and individual item scores are summed to obtain a composite score that ranges from zero to 12.

The Development of Composite Scales to Assess Attitudes Toward Stress Response and Recovery

Several new items were written specifically for this study to assess perceptions and attitudes related to stress response and recovery. The content of these items was informed by the stress-related attitudes and actions that the OSCAR program was designed to target. Perceptions and attitudes were rated on one of two five-point Likert scales, one with response options ranging from *strongly agree* to *strongly disagree* and the other with response options ranging from *not at all confident* to *completely confident*. All items were scored so that higher scores indicated more-positive (healthier) perceptions and attitudes toward stress response and recovery.

Some examples of these items include:

- I think I can handle additional deployments.

- I can recognize signs of stress in my fellow Marines.
- If I had a stress problem, I have buddies who would understand and help me get through it.
- I would be seen as weak if others knew I needed help with stress.

Because of the large number of items that were newly developed for this survey, we conducted an exploratory factor analysis[1] of item responses to determine if they could be combined to form a smaller number of interpretable factors. A total of 27 items were included in the exploratory factor analysis. Item responses were treated as categorical, using weighted least squares adjusted for means and variances estimation in Mplus, version 6.12. The rotation method was geomin, an oblique rotation method that allows the factors to correlate with each other. The eigenvalues, scree plot, and interpretability of each of the factor solutions were collectively taken into account to determine the final number of factors.

Based on the hypothesized factor structure, we considered solutions for between two and eight factors. According to the Kaiser criterion, in which all factors with eigenvalues greater than one are retained, a six-factor solution would have been chosen. Given concerns that the Kaiser criterion retains too many factors, however, we then looked to the scree plot to evaluate the tenability of a more parsimonious solution with a smaller number of factors. The scree plot, which shows the number of factors on the x-axis plotted against the eigenvalues on the y-axis, showed a dramatically steep decline—the steepest decline—after the first factor. The first eigenvalue was 8.4, followed by a marked decrease to the second eigenvalue of 2.5. The third eigenvalue was 1.9, and thereafter all eigenvalues were less than 1.5. Based on the scree plot, we assessed the potential viability of a two-factor solution, retaining only those factors with an eigenvalue greater than two.

The two-factor solution was subsequently examined for interpretability (i.e., the extent to which items loaded purely on a single factor) and correspondence with the hypothesized factor structure. Interpretability of the factor structure was maximized with a threshold of .45 or greater for interpretation of factor loadings. Four of the items did not load on any of the factors. Of the 23 remaining items, all items loaded on only one factor. The parsimonious two-factor solution proved highly interpretable and was therefore retained as the final solution. The first factor captured positive expectancies toward coping with and recovering from stress and comprised a total of 13 items. The second factor, which assessed perceived support for seeking help for stress problems from other Marines, comprised a total of ten items. Table B.1 shows the factor loadings for the two-factor solution.

---

[1] This was a common factor analysis.

Table B.1
Factor Loadings for the Final Two-Factor Solution Obtained in an Exploratory Factor Analysis of the Stress Attitudes Measure (N = 2,620)

Item/Factor	Factor Loadings	
	1	2
Factor 1: Positive expectancies toward coping with and recovering from stress		
Confident in your ability to help a buddy with stress	**.75**	−.03
Part of my job as a marine is to prevent stress reactions from getting out of hand for myself and my fellow marines.	**.70**	−.01
Confident in your ability to handle stress	**.65**	−.01
When I think a fellow marine is under too much stress, I know what to do.	**.64**	−.01
Everyone in our unit has a responsibility to help Marines cope with stress.	**.61**	.07
I am fully capable of doing my job in the unit.	**.60**	.05
It's possible to recover from a stress injury or illness and do your job as well as before.	**.53**	.02
I have seen buddies take care of stress problems successfully.	**.51**	.37
I can recognize signs of stress in my fellow marines.	**.50**	−.11
Confident that you could get helpful advice or information about stress if you needed it	**.50**	.30
Even the strongest marine can be affected by stress.	**.48**	−.04
If I had a stress problem, I have buddies who would understand and help me get through it.	**.48**	.33
I think I can handle additional deployments.	**.46**	.01
Factor 2: Perceived support for seeking help for stress problems from other marines		
I would be seen as weak if others knew I needed help with stress.	−.11	**.81**
If I sought help to deal with stress, my unit leadership might treat me differently.	−.12	**.74**
My leaders encourage seeking help for stress problems.	.14	**.62**
If I had a stress problem, I have leaders who would understand and help me get through it.	.39	**.58**
My leaders would commend me for getting help for a stress problem.	.00	**.56**
Members of my unit would have more confidence in me if I sought help for a stress problem.	−.02	**.54**
It would be too embarrassing to seek assistance for a stress problem.	.05	**.50**
I have seen leaders take care of stress problems successfully.	.43	**.50**
The Marine Corps supports those who have mental health problems.	.12	**.45**
Our leaders talk to us about their experiences with stress problems.	.23	**.45**

Table B.1—Continued

Item/Factor	Factor Loadings 1	2
Items that did not load on any factor		
A fellow marine's problems with stress are none of my business.	.29	.19
My buddies talk to each other about their experiences with stress problems.	.27	.18
Since I joined this unit there have been times when I have felt unable to do my job.	.44	.13
If I had a stress problem, I have a medical provider, chaplain, or corpsman who would understand and help me get through it.	.41	.38

NOTES: The factor loadings above, taken from the pattern matrix, reflect the unique relationship between the factor and the variable after accounting for variance shared with other factors. Only factor loadings greater than or equal to .45 were interpreted. The correspondence of items to the factor on which they load is indicated by a factor loading in bold font.

We assessed the internal consistency of composite scales composed of the items in each factor and found that both scales had good internal consistency (Chronbach's alpha for both = 0.83).

Statistical Analysis

Individuals are nested within companies, which are in turn nested within battalions. This implies a three-level data structure. However, because we did not have information on the company of many of the marines, we were unable to incorporate this level of clustering into our modeling strategy. Thus, we adjusted only for the clustering of observations within battalions in this set of analyses.

One of the battalions was surveyed at multiple time points prior to deployment. Because of high rates of turnover within this battalion between these time points, we treated these batches of survey respondents as separate battalions. As a result, our analyses include 15 clusters of respondents.

We also created poststratification sampling weights so that the weighted sociodemographic and service history characteristics of our sample would approximate those of the target population our survey findings are intended to generalize: active-duty and reserve marines of rank O6 or lower who deployed to Iraq or Afghanistan between March 2010 and December 2011. Sociodemographic and service history characteristics of the target population were determined using administrative data obtained from the DMDC. Characteristics on which the sampling weights were based included age, race/ethnicity, rank, marital status, parental status, and history of previous deployments to Iraq or Afghanistan. A raking algorithm (Bishop, Fienberg, and Holland,

1975; Deming, 1943) was used to construct the weights. Raking is a statistical procedure that uses an iterative process to obtain a set of weights that minimize the differences between the sample of marines that we surveyed and the broader population of marines who deployed during the same period on the demographic characteristics for which population values are known. The raking algorithm results in a set of sampling weights that allows our sample to closely approximate the target population on the set of demographic characteristics. Respondents who had missing data on one or more of the characteristics used to create the sampling weights were assigned a weight of one (n = 261). After applying the weights, the sample was nearly identical to the target population on the six sociodemographic and service history characteristics listed above.

APPENDIX C

Additional Results Tables

Table C.1
Current Stress/Mental Health Burden, by Battalion Type

	Infantry (n = 1,506)	Service Support (n = 1,114)
	Mean (95% CI)	
Lifetime severity of PTSD symptoms[a]	32.1 (30.5, 33.7)	31.8 (30.1, 33.5)
	Percentage (95% CI)	
MDD probable diagnosis (current)	12.3 (9.8, 14.8)	12.7 (9.5, 13.4)
High-risk drinking (current)	25.6 (20.9, 30.3)	25.7 (21.9, 29.5)
Perceived need of help with stress for self or buddy often or very often	19.6 (12.8, 26.4)	23.9 (16.1, 31.8)
Current stress continuum zone[b]		
Green (ready)	49.9 (44.5, 55.2)	44.8 (35.4, 54.2)
Yellow (reacting)	36.6 (32.9, 40.4)	40.6 (32.9, 48.2)
Orange (injured)	8.9 (6.2, 11.5)	10.9 (5.4, 16.4)
Red (ill)	1.9 (0.3, 3.5)	2.0 (0.4, 3.7)
Orange or red (versus green or yellow)	10.8 (6.8, 14.8)	13.0 (8.1, 17.8)

NOTE: All estimates in the table are weighted to be representative of all marines rank O6 or lower who deployed to Iraq or Afghanistan in 2010 or 2011.

[a] Lifetime severity of PTSD symptoms was assessed with a modified version of the 17-item PCL, in which respondents were asked to indicate the extent to which each symptom had been experienced "in your lifetime" instead of the standard time frame of the "past 30 days." Each symptom was rated on a scale that ranged from 1 (not at all) to 5 (extremely). Composite scale scores range from 17 to 85.

[b] Within columns, the percentages of respondents in different zones of the stress continuum sum to less than 100 percent due to missing data on this survey item.

Table C.2
Lifetime History of Potentially Traumatic Events, by Rank (N = 2,620)

	Mean (95% CI)		
	E1–E3 (n = 1,719)	**E4–E9 (n = 725)**	**Officer (n = 90)**
Average number of potentially traumatic events directly experienced[a,b,c,e]	3.5 (3.3, 3.8)	4.3 (3.8, 4.8)	2.9 (2.3, 3.5)
Types of potentially traumatic events directly experienced[f]		**Percent (95% CI)**	
Motor vehicle accident	64.3 (62.4, 66.1)	68.6 (61.7, 75.6)	64.0 (54.1, 73.9)
Sudden, unexpected death of a loved one[a,c,d]	48.6 (46.6, 50.6)	46.7 (41.9, 51.5)	29.3 (19.4, 39.2)
Other very stressful event	35.9 (31.7, 40.1)	41.5 (36.3, 46.7)	30.6 (19.6, 41.6)
Physical assault[a,c,d]	39.4 (36.1, 42.8)	39.9 (35.3, 44.4)	24.8 (13.5, 36.2)
Other serious accident[a,c,d]	30.0 (27.4, 32.4)	31.1 (26.6, 35.6)	16.7 (9.1, 24.3)
Natural disaster	26.3 (20.8, 31.8)	30.7 (22.3, 39.0)	24.1 (11.9, 36.4)
Combat[a,b,c]	6.5 (1.9, 11.3)	30.7 (22.9, 38.6)	12.3 (5.2, 19.4)
Fire/explosion	20.4 (18.2, 22.7)	28.9 (23.7, 34.2)	21.0 (7.6, 34.4)
Assault with a weapon	25.6 (22.4, 28.7)	24.8 (17.7, 31.9)	9.5 (0.1, 18.9)
Caused serious injury/death of another[a,c]	11.2 (7.7, 14.7)	17.3 (8.2, 26.4)	5.8 (0, 11.1)
Exposure to toxic substance[a,c,d]	11.5 (9.0, 14.0)	19.7 (13.9, 25.5)	4.6 (1.1, 8.0)
Witness violent death	8.2 (6.1, 10.4)	13.4 (6.8, 20.1)	6.1 (1.6, 10.7)
Life-threatening injury/illness	12.2 (9.5, 15.0)	14.8 (11.2, 18.3)	6.5 (0.9, 12.1)
Unwanted sexual experience other than sexual assault	4.6 (3.7, 5.5)	7.0 (2.7, 11.4)	9.5 (0.3, 18.8)
Severe human suffering	3.0 (1.6, 4.3)	3.5 (1.5, 5.5)	2.3 (–.02, 6.4)
Sexual assault	3.3 (2.1, 4.5)	5.4 (2.4, 8.3)	6.7 (–2.5, 15.8)
Captivity	1.6 (1.1, 2.0)	1.0 (0.2, 1.8)	0.6 (–0.4, 1.5)

NOTE: All estimates in the table are weighted to be representative of all marines who deployed to Iraq or Afghanistan in 2010 or 2011 of rank O6 or lower.

[a] Omnibus Rao-Scott chi-square test or adjusted Wald test is statistically significant at $p < .05$.

[b] The difference between respondents of rank E1–E3 and rank E4–E9 is statistically significant at $p < .05$.

[c] The difference between respondents of rank E4–E9 and officers is statistically significant at $p < .05$.

[d] The difference between respondents of rank E1–E3 and officers is statistically significant at $p < .05$.

[e] Participants were asked to indicate, for each of 17 traumatic events, whether they had directly experienced the event in their lifetime. The range of possible scores on this measure is 0 to 17. Cluster-adjusted Wald tests were conducted to determine whether there were significant differences by rank on the average number of potentially traumatic events experienced in one's lifetime.

[f] The Rao-Scott chi-square test was conducted to determine whether there were significant differences by rank in the percentage of respondents who reported having experienced each type of potentially traumatic event in their lifetime.

Table C.3
Lifetime History of Potentially Traumatic Events, by Battalion Type (N = 2,620)

	Mean (95% CI)	
	Infantry (n = 1,506)	**Service Support (n = 1,114)**
Average number of potentially traumatic events directly experienced[a,c]	4.2 (3.9, 4.5)	3.6 (3.3, 3.8)
Types of potentially traumatic events directly experienced[b]	**Percent (95% CI)**	
Motor vehicle accident	65.2 (59.2, 71.2)	67.4 (63.2, 71.6)
Sudden, unexpected death of a loved one	46.3 (41.8, 50.8)	44.7 (40.6, 48.8)
Other very stressful event[c]	40.7 (36.7, 44.6)	35.8 (32.7, 38.8)
Physical assault[c]	42.1 (38.5, 45.6)	34.4 (30.4, 38.3)
Other serious accident[c]	30.8 (28.9, 32.8)	27.4 (25.6, 29.2)
Natural disaster	31.7 (22.7, 40.7)	25.2 (19.3, 31.0)
Combat[c]	23.7 (18.9, 28.5)	15.2 (11.4, 19.0)
Fire/explosion	26.8 (21.3, 32.4)	22.8 (20.7, 24.9)
Assault with a weapon[c]	27.7 (24.3, 31.2)	19.5 (17.4, 21.6)
Caused serious injury/death of another[c]	19.9 (13.8, 26.0)	7.9 (5.2, 10.6)
Exposure to toxic substance[c]	17.3 (13.4, 21.3)	12.6 (9.8, 15.3)
Witness violent death[c]	14.2 (9.6, 18.8)	7.4 (5.2, 9.6)
Life-threatening injury/illness	14.2 (11.7, 16.6)	11.7 (9.1, 14.3)
Unwanted sexual experience other than sexual assault[c]	4.2 (3.0, 5.4)	8.3 (4.5, 12.1)
Severe human suffering[c]	4.8 (2.8, 6.7)	1.9 (0.4, 3.5)
Sexual assault[c]	2.7 (0.9, 4.6)	6.5 (4.4, 8.5)
Captivity[c]	1.8 (1.5, 2.1)	0.6 (0.3, 0.9)

NOTE: All estimates in the table are weighted to be representative of all marines who deployed to Iraq or Afghanistan in 2010 or 2011 of rank O6 or lower.

[a] Participants were asked to indicate, for each of 17 traumatic events, whether they had directly experienced the event in their lifetime. The range of possible scores on this measure is 0 to 17. Cluster-adjusted Wald tests were conducted to determine whether there were significant differences by rank on the average number of potentially traumatic events experienced in one's lifetime.

[b] The Rao-Scott chi-square test was conducted to determine whether there were significant differences by rank in the percentage of respondents who reported having experienced each type of potentially traumatic event in their lifetime.

[c] There is a statistically significant difference between battalion types at $p < .05$.

Table C.4
Help-Seeking Behaviors, by Battalion Type (N = 2,620)

	Percentage (95% CI)	
	Infantry (n = 1,506)	**Service Support (n = 1,114)**
Used help-seeking resources for stress, by type		
Buddy*	69.9 (66.6, 73.2)	73.8 (69.6, 77.9)
Leader*	44.6 (42.2, 47.0)	54.3 (48.0, 60.6)
Corpsman*	23.8 (21.3, 26.2)	16.1 (13.6, 18.6)
Chaplain*	16.2 (9.9, 22.6)	25.3 (21.9, 28.8)
Unit medical officer	11.8 (9.0, 14.5)	10.5 (7.8, 13.3)
Any	76.8 (72.2, 81.3)	81.5 (75.8, 87.3)
Recommended help-seeking resources for stress, by type		
Buddy	83.2 (78.6, 87.8)	84.7 (81.1, 88.2)
Leader*	64.0 (60.0, 68.0)	71.1 (64.7, 77.4)
Corpsman*	41.9 (37.1, 46.8)	32.7 (29.1, 36.3)
Chaplain	56.8 (48.8, 64.8)	63.9 (56.9, 71.0)
Unit medical officer	27.5 (19.3, 35.7)	29.1 (23.9, 34.3)
Any	87.8 (84.5, 91.2)	89.3 (85.1, 93.7)

NOTE: All estimates in the table are weighted to be representative of all marines who deployed to Iraq or Afghanistan in 2010 or 2011 of rank O6 or lower.

* There is a statistically significant difference between battalion types at $p < .05$.

Table C.5
Help-Seeking Behaviors, by Deployment History (N = 2,620)

	Percentage (95% CI)	
	Never Deployed (n = 1463)	Deployed Once or More (n = 1062)
Took action for stress most or all of the time*	57.3 (52.5, 62.2)	64.0 (58.6, 69.5)
Used help-seeking resources for stress, by type		
Buddy	72.5 (68.9, 76.0)	70.5 (64.9, 76.0)
Leader	49.9 (43.1, 56.7)	49.3 (43.1, 56.7)
Corpsman	19.4 (15.6, 23.1)	20.9 (17.8, 24.0)
Chaplain	20.5 (15.1, 26.0)	22.5 (16.9, 28.2)
Unit medical officer	10.4 (7.8, 13.0)	13.2 (10.1, 16.4)
Any	79.8 (74.5, 85.1)	77.8 (73.2, 82.5)
Recommended help-seeking resources for stress, by type		
Buddy	83.8 (80.4, 87.1)	84.9 (81.9, 87.9)
Leader*	66.4 (60.8, 72.0)	71.9 (67.0, 76.7)
Corpsman*	34.6 (29.7, 39.5)	44.5 (39.4, 49.7)
Chaplain*	57.1 (51.4, 62.9)	70.9 (63.8, 78.0)
Unit medical officer*	25.8 (20.4, 31.2)	35.9 (31.3, 40.6)
Any*	88.0 (84.8, 91.1)	91.0 (88.3, 93.6)

NOTE: All estimates in the table are weighted to be representative of all marines who deployed to Iraq or Afghanistan in 2010 or 2011 of rank O6 or lower.

* There is a statistically significant difference between marines with and without a history of previous deployments to Iraq or Afghanistan at $p < .05$.

Table C.6 Stress Response Attitudes in the Entire Sample (N = 2,620)

	Mean (95% CI)
Positive attitudes toward stress response and recovery[a]	4.01 (3.97, 4.05)
Confident in your ability to help a buddy with stress	3.55 (3.48, 3.62)
Part of my job as a Marine is to prevent stress reactions from getting out of hand for myself and my fellow Marines.	4.28 (4.19, 4.36)
Confident in your ability to handle stress	3.79 (3.72, 3.86)
When I think a fellow Marine is under too much stress, I know what to do.	3.78 (3.71, 3.85)
Everyone in our unit has a responsibility to help Marines cope with stress.	4.24 (4.14, 4.33)
I am fully capable of doing my job in the unit.	4.57 (4.50, 4.64)
It's possible to recover from a stress injury or illness and do your job as well as before.	4.19 (4.14, 4.24)
I have seen buddies take care of stress problems successfully.	3.67 (3.61, 3.73)
I can recognize signs of stress in my fellow marines	4.13 (4.09,4.18)
Confident that you could get helpful advice or information about stress if you needed it	3.55 (3.46, 3.63)
Even the strongest Marine can be affected by stress.	4.60, (4.53, 4.66)
If I had a stress problem, I have buddies who would understand and help me get through it.	3.89 (3.85, 3.94)
I think I can handle additional deployments.	3.92 (3.86, 3.99)
Perceived support for help-seeking from other Marines[a]	3.12 (3.06, 3.18)
I would be seen as weak if others knew I needed help with stress.[b]	3.11 (3.00, 3.23)
If I sought help to deal with stress, my unit leadership might treat me differently.[b]	3.07 (2.99, 3.16)
My leaders encourage seeking help for stress problems.	3.44 (3.37, 3.52)
If I had a stress problem, I have leaders who would understand and help me get through it.	3.61 (3.54, 3.69)
My leaders would commend me for getting help for a stress problem.	2.98 (2.89, 3.06)
Members of my unit would have more confidence in me if I sought help for a stress problem.	2.82 (2.70, 2.93)
It would be too embarrassing to seek assistance for a stress problem.[b]	2.72 (2.62, 2.81)
I have seen leaders take care of stress problems successfully.	3.49 (3.40, 3.57)
The Marine Corps supports those who have mental health problems.	3.21 (3.15, 3.27)
Our leaders talk to us about their experiences with stress problems.	2.54 (2.43, 2.64)

Table C.6—Continued

	Mean (95% CI)
Other items that were not included in either composite scale	
A fellow Marine's problems with stress are none of my business.	2.11 (2.03, 2.19)
My buddies talk to each other about their experiences with stress problems.	3.10 (3.04, 3.16)
Since I joined this unit there have been times when I have felt unable to do my job.	1.72 (1.62, 1.83)
If I had a stress problem, I have a medical provider, chaplain, or corpsman who would understand and help me get through it.	3.98 (3.90, 4.07)

NOTES: All estimates in the table are weighted to be representative of all marines who deployed to Iraq or Afghanistan in 2010 or 2011 of rank O6 or lower. The labels of the two composite scales that resulted from an exploratory factor analysis of stress response attitudes items are in bold font. The individual scale items that constitute each composite scale are indented in the rows underneath the scale label. Items that did not qualify for inclusion in either scale are listed under a third category in bold font called "Other items that were not included in either composite scale." Individual scale items were rated on a 5-point Likert scale with response options that ranged from 1 (strongly disagree) to 5 (strongly agree).

[a] Possible scores on the scales of positive expectancies toward coping with and recovering from stress and perceived support for help-seeking from marines range from 1 to 5, with higher scores indicating more positive, healthier attitudes.

[b] These individual scale items were reverse scored prior to computing the composite scale score for perceived support for help-seeking from marines.

Table C.7
Stress Response Attitudes, by Rank (N = 2,620)

	Mean (95% CI)		
	E1–E3 (n = 1,719)	E4–E9 (n = 725)	Officer (n = 90)
Positive attitudes toward stress response and recovery [a,b,d,e]	3.92 (3.86, 3.97)	4.06 (4.00, 4.13)	4.12 (4.02, 4.22)
Confident in your ability to help a buddy with stress[a,b]	3.45 (3.40, 3.50)	3.62 (3.52, 3.73)	3.56 (3.34, 3.79)
Part of my job as a Marine is to prevent stress reactions from getting out of hand for myself and my fellow Marines.[a,b,c,d]	4.09 (4.00, 4.18)	4.36 (4.24, 4.47)	4.57 (4.41, 4.73)
Confident in your ability to handle stress[a,b]	3.68 (3.57, 3.78)	3.88 (3.76, 3.97)	3.78 (3.59, 3.97)
When I think a fellow Marine is under too much stress, I know what to do.[a,b,d]	3.58 (3.48, 3.67)	3.91 (3.82, 4.00)	3.89 (3.73, 4.04)
Everyone in our unit has a responsibility to help Marines cope with stress.[a,c,d]	4.12 (4.00, 4.24)	4.26 (4.12, 4.40)	4.56 (4.37, 4.75)
I am fully capable of doing my job in the unit.[a,b]	4.50 (4.39, 4.60)	4.63 (4.52, 4.74)	4.58 (4.37, 4.78)
It's possible to recover from a stress injury or illness and do your job as well as before.[a,b,c,d]	4.07 (4.00, 4.13)	4.22 (4.16, 4.29)	4.49 (4.31, 4.67)
I have seen buddies take care of stress problems successfully.	3.65 (3.56, 3.75)	3.67 (3.61, 3.73)	3.67 (3.44, 3.91)
I can recognize signs of stress in my fellow Marines[a,b,d]	4.06 (4.02, 4.11)	4.18 (4.10, 4.27)	4.16 (4.07, 4.24)
Confident that you could get helpful advice or information about stress if you needed it[a,b]	3.42 (3.33, 3.50)	3.64 (3.53, 3.75)	3.57 (3.15, 3.98)
Even the strongest Marine can be affected by stress.	4.56 (4.51, 4.61)	4.61 (4.52, 4.71)	4.66 (4.55, 4.77)
If I had a stress problem, I have buddies who would understand and help me get through it.	3.93 (3.85, 4.00)	3.86 (3.77, 3.94)	3.95 (3.83, 4.07)
I think I can handle additional deployments.[a,b]	3.81 (3.74, 3.88)	3.98 (3.86, 4.10)	4.04 (3.80, 4.27)
Perceived support for help-seeking from other Marines[e]	3.10 (3.01, 3.19)	3.12 (3.04, 3.21)	3.15 (2.94, 3.36)
I would be seen as weak if others knew needed help with stress.[a,c,d,f]	3.12 (2.96, 3.28)	3.04 (2.89, 3.20)	3.41 (3.19, 3.64)
If I sought help to deal with stress, my unit leadership might treat me differently.[f]	3.08 (2.99, 3.17)	3.06 (2.94, 3.18)	3.12 (2.73, 3.52)
My leaders encourage seeking help for stress problems.	3.41 (3.32, 3.50)	3.46 (3.31, 3.62)	3.47 (3.22, 3.71)
If I had a stress problem, I have leaders who would understand and help me get through it.	3.64 (3.47, 3.81)	3.56 (3.43, 3.69)	3.74 (3.47, 4.00)

Table C.7—Continued

	Mean (95% CI)		
	E1–E3 (n = 1,719)	E4–E9 (n = 725)	Officer (n = 90)
My leaders would commend me for getting help for a stress problem.	2.97 (2.87, 3.06)	2.96 (2.85, 3.08)	3.07 (2.82, 3.33)
Members of my unit would have more confidence in me if I sought help for a stress problem.[a,b,c,d]	2.94 (2.83, 3.04)	2.79 (2.63, 2.94)	2.51 (2.25, 2.76)
It would be too embarrassing to seek assistance for a stress problem.[a,b,f]	2.78 (2.69, 2.88)	2.64 (2.52, 2.77)	2.82 (2.43, 3.21)
I have seen leaders take care of stress problems successfully.	3.46 (3.33, 3.59)	3.46 (3.37, 3.56)	3.69 (3.42, 3.96)
The Marine Corps supports those who have mental health problems.[a,c,d]	3.10 (2.97, 3.23)	3.21 (3.12, 3.30)	3.62 (3.40, 3.84)
Our leaders talk to us about their experiences with stress problems.	2.50 (2.39, 2.61)	2.56 (2.41, 2.71)	2.56 (2.30, 2.82)
Other items that were not included in either composite scale			
A fellow Marine's problems with stress are none of my business.[a,b,d]	2.29 (2.23, 2.36)	2.02 (1.87, 2.18)	1.87 (1.63, 2.10)
My buddies talk to each other about their experiences with stress problems.	3.13 (3.03, 3.22)	3.10 (2.99, 3.21)	2.99 (2.83, 3.14)
Since I joined this unit there have been times when I have felt unable to do my job.[a,c,d]	1.80 (1.66, 1.94)	1.71 (1.60, 1.82)	1.51 (1.31, 1.71)
If I had a stress problem, I have a medical provider, chaplain, or corpsman who would understand and help me get through it.	3.94 (3.85, 4.04)	4.02 (3.89, 4.14)	3.97 (3.72, 4.23)

NOTES: All estimates in the table are weighted to be representative of all marines who deployed to Iraq or Afghanistan in 2010 or 2011 of rank O6 or lower. The labels of the two composite scales that resulted from an exploratory factor analysis of items designed to assess stress response attitudes are in bold font. The individual scale items that constitute each composite scale are indented in the rows underneath the scale label. Items that did not qualify for inclusion in either scale are listed under a third category in bold font called "Other items that were not included in either composite scale." Individual scale items were rated on a Likert scale with response options that ranged from 1 (strongly disagree) to 5 (strongly agree).

[a] Omnibus cluster-adjusted Wald joint test is statistically significant at $p < .05$.

[b] Difference between respondents of rank E1–E3 and rank E4–E9 is statistically significant at $p < .05$.

[c] Difference between respondents of rank E4–E9 and officers is statistically significant at $p < .05$.

[d] Difference between respondents of rank E1–E3 and officers is statistically significant at $p < .05$.

[e] Possible scores on the scales of positive expectancies toward coping with and recovering from stress and perceived support for help-seeking from Marines range from 1 to 5, with higher scores indicating more positive, healthier attitudes.

[f] These individual scale items were reverse scored prior to computing the composite scale score for perceived support for help-seeking from marines.

Table C.8
Stress Response Attitudes, by Deployment History (N= 2,620)

	Mean (95% CI)	
	Never Deployed (n= 1,463)	**Deployed Once or More (n= 1,062)**
Positive attitudes toward stress response and recovery[a]*	3.98 (3.94, 4.03)	4.10 (4.04, 4.16)
Confident in your ability to help a buddy with stress*	3.50 (3.42, 3.57)	3.71 (3.61, 3.81)
Part of my job as a Marine is to prevent stress reactions from getting out of hand for myself and my fellow Marines.*	4.24 (4.16, 4.33)	4.37 (4.27, 4.48)
Confident in your ability to handle stress*	3.75 (3.67, 3.84)	3.90 (3.81, 3.99)
When I think a fellow Marine is under too much stress, I know what to do.*	3.71 (3.63, 3.80)	3.97 (3.87, 4.07)
Everyone in our unit has a responsibility to help Marines cope with stress.	4.23 (4.12, 4.34)	4.26 (4.14, 4.38)
I am fully capable of doing my job in the unit.*	4.54 (4.46, 4.62)	4.67 (4.59, 4.74)
It's possible to recover from a stress injury or illness and do your job as well as before.	4.18 (4.13, 4.24)	4.21 (4.13, 4.30)
I have seen buddies take care of stress problems successfully.	3.64 (3.56, 3.71)	3.74 (3.67, 3.82)
I can recognize signs of stress in my fellow marines*	4.11 (4.06, 4.16)	4.21 (4.14, 4.27)
Confident that you could get helpful advice or information about stress if you needed it*	3.51 (3.41, 3.62)	3.65 (3.52, 3.77)
Even the strongest Marine can be affected by stress.*	4.58 (4.51, 4.65)	4.65 (4.58, 4.72)
If I had a stress problem, I have buddies who would understand and help me get through it.	3.90 (3.85, 3.96)	3.87 (3.79, 3.95)
I think I can handle additional deployments.*	3.86 (3.78, 3.94)	4.07 (3.97, 4.17)
Perceived support for help-seeking from other Marines[a]	3.11 (3.05, 3.17)	3.14 (3.05, 3.24)
I would be seen as weak if others knew I needed help with stress.[b]*	3.15 (3.03, 3.28)	3.00 (2.85, 3.14)
If I sought help to deal with stress, my unit leadership might treat me differently.[b]	3.09 (2.99, 3.20)	3.01 (2.87, 3.16)
My leaders encourage seeking help for stress problems.	3.45 (3.37, 3.53)	3.43 (3.32, 3.55)
If I had a stress problem, I have leaders who would understand and help me get through it.	3.64 (3.55, 3.72)	3.54 (3.40, 3.67)
My leaders would commend me for getting help for a stress problem.	2.97 (2.89, 3.06)	2.98 (2.81, 3.15)

Table C.8—Continued

	Mean (95% CI)	
	Never Deployed (n= 1,463)	**Deployed Once or More (n= 1,062)**
Members of my unit would have more confidence in me if I sought help for a stress problem.	2.82 (2.70, 2.94)	2.80 (2.66, 2.95)
It would be too embarrassing to seek assistance for a stress problem.[b]	2.73 (2.62, 2.85)	2.67 (2.59, 2.75)
I have seen leaders take care of stress problems successfully.	3.47 (3.37, 3.58)	3.52 (3.43, 3.60)
The Marine Corps supports those who have mental health problems.*	3.17 (3.11, 3.23)	3.32 (3.14, 3.50)
Our leaders talk to us about their experiences with stress problems.	2.53 (2.42, 2.65)	2.54 (2.41, 2.67)
Other items that were not included in either composite scale		
A fellow Marine's problems with stress are none of my business.*	2.19 (2.10, 2.27)	1.90 (1.80, 2.00)
My buddies talk to each other about their experiences with stress problems.	3.09 (3.02, 3.16)	3.11 (3.02, 3.20)
Since I joined this unit there have been times when I have felt unable to do my job.*	1.77 (1.64, 1.90)	1.59 (1.48, 1.70)
If I had a stress problem, I have a medical provider, chaplain, or corpsman who would understand and help me get through it.	3.99 (3.90, 4.08)	3.97 (3.85, 4.09)

NOTES: All estimates in the table are weighted to be representative of all marines who deployed to Iraq or Afghanistan in 2010 or 2011 of rank O6 or lower. The labels of the two composite scales that resulted from an exploratory factor analysis of items designed to assess stress response attitudes are in bold font. The individual scale items that constitute each composite scale are indented in the rows underneath the scale label. Items that did not qualify for inclusion in either scale are listed under a third category in bold font called "Other items that were not included in either composite scale." Individual scale items were rated on a Likert scale with response options that ranged from 1 (strongly disagree) to 5 (strongly agree). Asterisks denote statistical significance of the cluster-adjusted Wald test at $p < .05$.

[a] Possible scores on the scales of positive expectancies toward coping with and recovering from stress and perceived support for help-seeking from Marines range from 1 to 5, with higher scores indicating more positive, healthier attitudes.

[b] These individual scale items were reverse scored prior to computing the composite scale score for perceived support for help-seeking from marines.

Table C.9
Stress Response Attitudes, by Battalion Type (N = 2,620)

	Mean (95% CI)	
	Infantry (n = 1,506)	**Service Support (n = 1,114)**
Positive attitudes toward stress response and recovery [a]	4.00 (3.96, 4.05)	4.02 (3.96, 4.08)
Confident in your ability to help a buddy with stress	3.51 (3.44, 3.57)	3.59 (3.51, 3.67)
Part of my job as a Marine is to prevent stress reactions from getting out of hand for myself and my fellow Marines.	4.24 (4.15, 4.33)	4.30 (4.19, 4.41)
Confident in your ability to handle stress	3.81 (3.71, 3.91)	3.77 (3.68, 3.87)
When I think a fellow Marine is under too much stress, I know what to do.	3.77 (3.65, 3.89)	3.78 (3.71, 3.86)
Everyone in our unit has a responsibility to help Marines cope with stress.	4.22 (4.10, 4.35)	4.25 (4.11, 4.39)
I am fully capable of doing my job in the unit.	4.54 (4.45, 4.64)	4.60 (4.50, 4.69)
It's possible to recover from a stress injury or illness and do your job as well as before.	4.21 (4.14, 4.28)	4.21 (4.10, 4.25)
I have seen buddies take care of stress problems successfully.	3.70 (3.63, 3.78)	3.63 (3.54, 3.72)
I can recognize signs of stress in my fellow marines.	4.15 (4.11, 4.18)	4.13 (4.04, 4.21)
Confident that you could get helpful advice or information about stress if you needed it	3.50 (3.40, 3.59)	3.59 (3.47, 3.71)
Even the strongest Marine can be affected by stress.*	4.54 (4.50, 4.59)	4.64 (4.59, 4.70)
If I had a stress problem, I have buddies who would understand and help me get through it.	3.90 (3.86, 3.94)	3.89 (3.81, 3.97)
I think I can handle additional deployments.	3.95 (3.85, 4.04)	3.90 (3.80, 3.99)
Perceived support for help-seeking from other Marines[a]	3.09 (3.02, 3.17)	3.14 (3.07, 3.22)
I would be seen as weak if others knew I needed help with stress.[b]*	3.20 (3.06, 3.33)	3.03 (2.91, 3.16)
If I sought help to deal with stress, my unit leadership might treat me differently.[b]*	3.12 (3.01, 3.23)	3.03 (2.93, 3.13)
My leaders encourage seeking help for stress problems.	3.41 (3.34, 3.48)	3.48 (3.37, 3.58)
If I had a stress problem, I have leaders who would understand and help me get through it.	3.63 (3.56, 3.70)	3.59 (3.47, 3.72)
My leaders would commend me for getting help for a stress problem.	2.94 (2.81, 3.08)	3.01 (2.90, 3.11)
Members of my unit would have more confidence in me if I sought help for a stress problem.	2.80 (2.62, 2.98)	2.83 (2.69, 2.97)

Table C.9—Continued

	Mean (95% CI)	
	Infantry (n = 1,506)	**Service Support (n = 1,114)**
It would be too embarrassing to seek assistance for a stress problem.[b]*	2.77 (2.69, 2.86)	2.67 (2.54, 2.80)
I have seen leaders take care of stress problems successfully.	3.57 (3.46, 3.67)	3.41 (3.29, 3.53)
The Marine Corps supports those who have mental health problems.	3.17 (3.08, 3.26)	3.25 (3.19, 3.30)
Our leaders talk to us about their experiences with stress problems.	2.52 (2.41, 2.62)	2.55 (2.38, 2.72)
Other items that were not included in either composite scale		
A fellow Marine's problems with stress are none of my business.*	2.19 (2.12, 2.27)	2.04 (2.00, 2.08)
My buddies talk to each other about their experiences with stress problems.	3.09 (3.04, 3.15)	3.10 (3.00, 3.21)
Since I joined this unit there have been times when I have felt unable to do my job.*	1.67 (1.57, 1.77)	1.77 (1.62, 1.93)
If I had a stress problem, I have a medical provider, chaplain, or corpsman who would understand and help me get through it.	3.97 (3.88, 4.07)	3.99 (3.86, 4.12)

NOTES: All estimates in the table are weighted to be representative of all marines who deployed to Iraq or Afghanistan in 2010 or 2011 of rank O6 or lower. The labels of the two composite scales that resulted from an exploratory factor analysis of items designed to assess stress response attitudes are in bold font. The individual scale items that constitute each composite scale are indented in the rows underneath the scale label. Items that did not qualify for inclusion in either scale are listed under a third category in bold font called "Other items that were not included in either composite scale." Individual scale items were rated on a Likert scale with response options that ranged from 1 (strongly disagree) to 5 (strongly agree). Asterisks denote statistical significance of the cluster-adjusted Wald test at $p < .05$.

[a] Possible scores on the scales of positive expectancies toward coping with and recovering from stress and perceived support for help-seeking from Marines range from 1 to 5, with higher scores indicating more positive, healthier attitudes.

[b] These individual scale items were reverse scored prior to computing the composite scale score for perceived support for help-seeking from marines.

References

American Psychiatric Association, *Diagnostic and Statistical Manual of Mental Disorder*, 4th ed., Washington, D.C.: American Psychiatric Association, 1994.

Bishop, Y. M. M., S. E. Fienberg, and P. W. Holland, *Discrete Multivariate Analysis: Theory and Practice*, Cambridge, Mass.: MIT Press, 1975.

Bliese, Paul D., Kathleen M. Wright, Amy B. Adler, Jeffrey L. Thomas, and Charles W. Hoge, "Timing of Postcombat Mental Health Assessments," *Psychological Services*, Vol. 4, No. 3, 2007, pp. 141–148.

Bush, K., D. R. Kivlahan, M. B. McDonell, S. D. Fihn, and K. A. Bradley, "The AUDIT Alcohol Consumption Questions (AUDIT-C): An Effective Brief Screening Test for Problem Drinking. Ambulatory Care Quality Improvement Project (ACQUIP) Alcohol Use Disorders Identification Test," *Archives of Internal Medicine*, Vol. 158, No. 16, 1998, pp. 1789–1795.

Clancy, Carolina P., Anna Graybeal, Whitney P. Tompson, Kourtni S. Badgett, Michelle E. Feldman, Patrick S. Calhoun, Alaattin Erkanli, Michael A. Hertzberg, and Jean C. Beckham, "Lifetime Trauma Exposure in Veterans with Military-Related Post-Traumatic Stress Disorder: Association with Current Sympatomatology," *Journal of Clinical Psychiatry*, Vol. 67, 2006, pp. 1346–1353.

Dawson, Deborah A., "Effectiveness of the Derived Alcohol Use Disorders Identification Test (AUDIT-C) in Screening for Alcohol Use Disorders and Risk Drinking in the U.S. General Population," *Alcoholism: Clinical & Experimental Research*, Vol. 29, No. 5, 2005, pp. 844–854.

Deming, W. E., *Statistical Adjustment of Data*, New York: Wiley, 1943.

Eisen, Susan V., Mark R. Schultz, Dawne Vogt, Mark E. Glickman, A. Rani Elwy, Mari-Lynn Drainoni, Princess E. Osei-Bonsu, and James Martin, "Mental and Physical Health Status and Alcohol and Drug Use Following Return from Deployment to Iraq or Afghanistan," *American Journal of Public Health*, Vol. 102, No. S1, 2012, pp. S66–S73.

Gray, Matt J., Brett T. Litz, Julie L. Hsu, and Thomas W. Lombardo, "Psychometric Properties of the Life Events Checklist," *Assessment*, Vol. 11, No. 4, 2004, pp. 330–341.

Greden, John F., Marcia Valenstein, Jane Spinner, Adrian Blow, Lisa A. Gorman, Gregory W. Dalack, Sheila Marcus, and Michelle Kees, "Buddy-to-Buddy, a Citizen Soldier Peer Support Program to Counteract Stigma, PTSD, Depression, and Suicide," *Annals of the New York Academy of Sciences*, Vol. 1208, No. 1, 2010, pp. 90–97.

Hawkins, Eric J., Gwendolyn T. Lapham, Daniel R. Kivlahan, and Katharine A. Bradley, "Recognition and Management of Alcohol Misuse in OEF/OIF and Other Veterans in the VA: A Cross-Sectional Study," *Drug and Alcohol Dependence*, Vol. 109, No. 1-3, 2010, pp. 147–153.

Hoge, Charles W., Jennifer L. Auchterlonie, and Charles S. Milliken, "Mental Health Problems, Use of Mental Health Services, and Attrition from Military Service After Returning from Deployment to Iraq or Afghanistan," *JAMA: The Journal of the American Medical Association*, Vol. 295, No. 9, 2006, pp. 1023–1032.

Hoge, Charles W., Carl A. Castro, Stephen C. Messer, Dennis McGurk, Dave I. Cotting, and Robert L. Koffman, "Combat Duty in Iraq and Afghanistan, Mental Health Problems, and Barriers to Care," *New England Journal of Medicine*, Vol. 351, No. 1, 2004, pp. 13–22.

Hourani, Laurel L., Huixing Yuan, and Robert M. Bray, "Psychosocial and Health Correlates of Types of Traumatic Event Exposures Among U.S. Military Personnel," *Military Medicine*, Vol. 168, No. 9, 2003, pp. 737–743.

HR 2647, "National Defense Authorization Act for Fiscal Year 2010: Section 708—Mental Health Assessments for Members of the Armed Forces Deployed in Connection with a Contingency Operation," 111th Congress, 1st Session, 2009.

Institute of Medicine, *Returning Home from Iraq and Afghanistan: Preliminary Assessment of Readjustment Needs of Veterans, Service Members, and Their Families*, Washington, D.C.: The National Academies Press, 2010.

———, *Treatment for Posttraumatic Stress Disorder in Military and Veteran Populations: Initial Assessment*, Washington, D.C.: The National Academies Press, 2012.

J-MHAT 7 OEF, "Joint Mental Health Advisory Team 7 (J-MHAT 7) Operation Enduring Freedom 2010 Afghanistan," 2011. As of September 17, 2012:
http://www.armymedicine.army.mil/reports/mhat/mhat_vii/J_MHAT_7.pdf

Kessler, Ronald C., "Posttraumatic Stress Disorder: The Burden to the Individual and to Society," *The Journal of Clinical Psychiatry*, Vol. 61 Suppl. 5, 2000, pp. 4–12.

Kessler, Ronald C., Amanda Sonnega, Evelyn Bromet, Michael Hughes, and Christopher B. Nelson, "Posttraumatic Stress Disorder in the National Comorbidity Survey," *Archives of General Psychiatry*, Vol. 52, No. 12, 1995, pp. 1048–1060.

Kroenke, Kurt, Robert L. Spitzer, and Janet B. W. Williams, "The PHQ-9: Validity of a Brief Depression Severity Measure," *Journal of General Internal Medicine*, Vol. 16, No. 9, 2001, pp. 606–613.

———, "The Patient Health Questionnaire-2: Validity of a Two-Item Depression Screener," *Medical Care*, Vol. 41, No. 11, 2003, pp. 1284–1292.

Kroenke, Kurt, Tara W. Strine, Robert L. Spitzer, Janet B. W. Williams, Joyce T. Berry, and Ali H. Mokdad, "The PHQ-8 as a Measure of Current Depression in the General Population," *Journal of Affective Disorders*, Vol. 114, No. 1-3, 2009, pp. 163–173.

Lapierre, Coady B., Andria F. Schwegler, and Bill J. LaBauve, "Posttraumatic Stress and Depression Symptoms in Soldiers Returning from Combat Operations in Iraq and Afghanistan," *Journal of Traumatic Stress*, Vol. 20, No. 6, 2007, pp. 933–943.

Löwe, Bernd, Kurt Kroenke, Wolfgang Herzog, and Kerstin Gräfe, "Measuring Depression Outcome with a Brief Self-Report Instrument: Sensitivity to Change of the Patient Health Questionnaire (PHQ-9)," *Journal of Affective Disorders*, Vol. 81, No. 1, 2004, pp. 61–66.

Maguen, Shira, Li Ren, Jeane O. Bosch, Charles R. Marmar, and Karen H. Seal, "Gender Differences in Mental Health Diagnoses Among Iraq and Afghanistan Veterans Enrolled in Veterans Affairs Health Care," *American Journal of Public Health*, Vol. 100, No. 12, 2010, pp. 2450–2456.

The Management of Substance Use Disorders Working Group, VA/DoD Clinical Practice Guideline for Management of Substance Use Disorders (SUD), 2009. As of May 9, 2013: http://www.healthquality.va.gov/sud/sud_full_601f.pdf

McLay, R. N., W. E. Deal, J. A. Murphy, K. B. Center, T. T. Kolkow, and T. A. Grieger, "On-the-Record Screenings Versus Anonymous Surveys in Reporting PTSD," *The American Journal of Psychiatry*, Vol. 165, No. 6, 2008, pp. 775–776.

Milliken, Charles S., Jennifer L. Auchterlonie, and Charles W. Hoge, "Longitudinal Assessment of Mental Health Problems Among Active and Reserve Component Soldiers Returning from the Iraq War," *JAMA: The Journal of the American Medical Association*, Vol. 298, No. 18, 2007, pp. 2141–2148.

Nash, William P., and Patricia J. Watson, "Review of VA/DOD Clinical Practice Guideline on Management of Acute Stress and Interventions to Prevent Posttraumatic Stress Disorder," *Journal of Rehabilitation Research and Development*, Vol. 49, No. 5, 2012, pp. 637–648.

NCCOSC, "5 Core Leadership Functions," Naval Center for Combat and Operational Stress Control, undated. As of September 17, 2012: http://www.med.navy.mil/sites/nmcsd/nccosc/leadersV2/infoAndTools/5CoreLeadershipFunctions/Pages/default.aspx

Phillips, Christopher J., Cynthia A. Leardmann, Gia R. Gumbs, and Besa Smith, "Risk Factors for Posttraumatic Stress Disorder Among Deployed U.S. Male Marines," *BMC Psychiatry*, Vol. 10, 2010, p. 52.

Ramchand, Rajeev, Benjamin R. Karney, Karen Chan Osilla, Rachel M. Burns, and Leah Barnes Caldarone, "Prevalence of PTSD, Depression, and TBI Among Returning Service members," in Terri Tanielian and Lisa H. Jaycox, eds., *Invisible Wounds of War: Psychological and Cognitive Injuries, Their Consequences, and Services to Assist Recovery*, Santa Monica, Calif.: RAND Corporation, MG-720-CCF, 2008, pp. 35–85. As of August 8, 2012: http://www.rand.org/pubs/monographs/MG720

Ramchand, Rajeev, Jeremy Miles, Terry Schell, Lisa Jaycox, Grant N. Marshall, and Terri Tanielian, "Prevalence and Correlates of Drinking Behaviors Among Previously Deployed Military and Matched Civilian Populations," *Military Psychology*, Vol. 23, No. 1, 2011, pp. 6–21.

Ramchand, Rajeev, Terry L. Schell, Benjamin R. Karney, Karen Chan Osilla, Rachel M. Burns, and Leah Barnes Caldarone, "Disparate Prevalence Estimates of PTSD Among Service Members Who Served in Iraq and Afghanistan: Possible Explanations," *Journal of Traumatic Stress*, Vol. 23, No. 1, 2010, pp. 59–68.

Ruggiero, Kenneth J., Kevin Del Ben, Joseph R. Scotti, and Aline E. Rabalais, "Psychometric Properties of the PTSD Checklist—Civilian Version," *Journal of Traumatic Stress*, Vol. 16, No. 5, 2003, p. 495.

Sandweiss, Donald A., Donald J. Slymen, Cynthia A. Leardmann, Besa Smith, Martin R. White, Edward J. Boyko, Tomoko I. Hooper, Gary D. Gackstetter, Paul J. Amoroso, and Tyler C. Smith, "Preinjury Psychiatric Status, Injury Severity, and Postdeployment Posttraumatic Stress Disorder," *Archives of General Psychiatry*, Vol. 68, No. 5, 2011, pp. 496–504.

Schell, Terry L., and Grant N. Marshall, "Survey of Individuals Previously Deployed for OEF/OIF," in Terri Tanielian and Lisa H. Jaycox, eds., *Invisible Wounds of War: Psychological and Cognitive Injuries, Their Consequences, and Services to Assist Recovery,* Santa Monica, Calif.: RAND Corporation, MG-720-CCF, 2008, pp. 87–115. As of August 8, 2012: http://www.rand.org/pubs/monographs/MG720

Seal, Karen H., Thomas J. Metzler, Kristian S. Gima, Daniel Bertenthal, Shira Maguen, and Charles R. Marmar, "Trends and Risk Factors for Mental Health Diagnoses Among Iraq and Afghanistan Veterans Using Department of Veterans Affairs Health Care, 2002–2008," *American Journal of Public Health*, Vol. 99, No. 9, 2009, pp. 1651–1658.

Shen, Yu-Chu, Jeremy Arkes, and Thomas V. Williams, "Effects of Iraq/Afghanistan Deployments on Major Depression and Substance Use Disorder: Analysis of Active Duty Personnel in the U.S. Military," *American Journal of Public Health*, Vol. 102, No. S1, 2012, pp. S80–S87.

Smith, Tyler C., Margaret A. K. Ryan, Deborah L. Wingard, Donald J. Slymen, James F. Sallis, and Donna Kritz-Silverstein, "New-Onset and Persistent Symptoms of Post-Traumatic Stress Disorder Self Reported After Deployment and Combat Exposures: Prospective Population Based U.S. Military Cohort Study," *BMJ: British Medical Journal (International Edition)*, Vol. 336, No. 7640, 2008, pp. 366–371.

Sundin, J., N. T. Fear, A. Iversen, R. J. Rona, and S. Wessely, "PTSD After Deployment to Iraq: Conflicting Rates, Conflicting Claims," *Psychological Medicine: A Journal of Research in Psychiatry and the Allied Sciences*, Vol. 40, No. 3, 2010, pp. 367–382.

Tanielian, Terri, and Lisa H. Jaycox, eds., *Invisible Wounds of War: Psychological and Cognitive Injuries, Their Consequences, and Services to Assist Recovery*, Santa Monica, Calif.: RAND Corporation, MG-720-CCF, 2008. As of August 8, 2012:
http://www.rand.org/pubs/monographs/MG720

Thomas, Jeffrey L., Joshua E. Wilk, Lyndon A. Riviere, Dennis McGurk, Carl A. Castro, and Charles W. Hoge, "Prevalence of Mental Health Problems and Functional Impairment Among Active Component and National Guard Soldiers 3 and 12 Months Following Combat in Iraq," *Archives of General Psychiatry*, Vol. 67, No. 6, 2010, pp. 614–623.

U.S. Marine Corps, "Combat and Operational Stress Control," Marine Corps Reference Publication (MCRP) 6-11C and Navy Tactics, Techniques, and Procedures (NTTP) 1-15M, 2010. As of September 17, 2012:
http://www.uscg.mil/worklife/docs/pdf/Navy_and_Marine_Corps_OSC_Doctrine_Dec_2010%5b1%5d.pdf

Vaughan, Christine Anne, Terry L. Schell, Lisa H. Jaycox, Grant N. Marshall, and Terri Tanielian, "Quantitative Needs Assessment of New York State Veterans and Their Spouses," in Terry L. Schell and Terri Tanielian, eds., *A Needs Assessment of New York State Veterans: Final Report to the New York State Health Foundation*, Santa Monica, Calif.: RAND Corporation, TR-920-NYSHF, 2011. As of August 29, 2012:
http://www.rand.org/pubs/technical_reports/TR920

Warner, Christopher H., George N. Appenzeller, Thomas Grieger, Slava Belenkiy, Jill Breitbach, Jessica Parker, Carolynn M. Warner, and Charles Hoge, "Importance of Anonymity to Encourage Honest Reporting in Mental Health Screening After Combat Deployment," *Archives of General Psychiatry*, Vol. 68, No. 10, 2011a, pp. 1063–1071.

———, "Effectiveness of Mental Health Screening and Coordination of In-Theater Care Prior to Deployment to Iraq: A Cohort Study," *American Journal of Psychiatry*, Vol. 168, No. 4, 2011b, pp. 378–385.

Weathers, F. W., B. T. Litz, D. S. Herman, J. A. Huska, and T. M. Keane, "The PTSD Checklist (PCL): Reliability, Validity, and Diagnostic Utility," paper presented at the International Society for Traumatic Stress Studies, San Antonio, Tex., 1993.

Weinick, Robin M., Ellen Burke Beckjord, Carrie M. Farmer, Laurie T. Martin, Emily M. Gillen, Joie Acosta, Michael P. Fisher, Jeffrey Garnett, Gabriella C. Gonzalez, Todd C. Helmus, Lisa H. Jaycox, Kerry Reynolds, Nicholas Salcedo, and Deborah M. Scharf, *Programs Addressing Psychological Health and Traumatic Brain Injury Among U.S. Military Service Members and Their Families*, Santa Monica, Calif.: RAND Corporation, TR-950-OSD, 2011. As of August 8, 2012: http://www.rand.org/pubs/technical_reports/TR950

Wilk, Joshua E., Paul D. Bliese, Paul Y. Kim, Jeffrey L. Thomas, Dennis McGurk, and Charles W. Hoge, "Relationship of Combat Experiences to Alcohol Misuse Among U.S. Soldiers Returning from the Iraq War," *Drug & Alcohol Dependence*, Vol. 108, No. 1/2, 2010, pp. 115–121.

Wright, Kathleen M., Oscar A. Cabrera, Rachel D. Eckford, Amy B. Adler, and Paul D. Bliese, "The Impact of Predeployment Functional Impairment on Mental Health After Combat," *Psychological Trauma: Theory, Research, Practice, and Policy*, 2011.